D1569561

Becoming a
BREAST CANCER NURSE NAVIGATOR

Lillie D. Shockney, RN, BS, MAS

Administrative Director
Johns Hopkins Avon Foundation Comprehensive Breast Center
University Distinguished Service Associate Professor of Breast Cancer
Associate Professor, Departments of Surgery and Gynecology
Johns Hopkins University School of Medicine
Associate Professor
Johns Hopkins University School of Nursing
Baltimore, Maryland

JONES AND BARTLETT PUBLISHERS
Sudbury, Massachusetts
BOSTON   TORONTO   LONDON   SINGAPORE

World Headquarters

Jones and Bartlett Publishers	Jones and Bartlett Publishers	Jones and Bartlett Publishers
40 Tall Pine Drive	Canada	International
Sudbury, MA 01776	6339 Ormindale Way	Barb House, Barb Mews
978-443-5000	Mississauga, Ontario L5V 1J2	London W6 7PA
info@jbpub.com	Canada	United Kingdom
www.jbpub.com		

Jones and Bartlett's books and products are available through most bookstores and online booksellers. To contact Jones and Bartlett Publishers directly, call 800-832-0034, fax 978-443-8000, or visit our website, www.jbpub.com.

Substantial discounts on bulk quantities of Jones and Bartlett's publications are available to corporations, professional associations, and other qualified organizations. For details and specific discount information, contact the special sales department at Jones and Bartlett via the above contact information or send an email to specialsales@jbpub.com.

The authors, editor, and publisher have made every effort to provide accurate information. However, they are not responsible for errors, omissions, or for any outcomes related to the use of the contents of this book and take no responsibility for the use of the products and procedures described. Treatments and side effects described in this book may not be applicable to all people; likewise, some people may require a dose or experience a side effect that is not described herein. Drugs and medical devices are discussed that may have limited availability controlled by the Food and Drug Administration (FDA) for use only in a research study or clinical trial. Research, clinical practice, and government regulations often change the accepted standard in this field. When consideration is being given to use of any drug in the clinical setting, the health care provider or reader is responsible for determining FDA status of the drug, reading the package insert, and reviewing prescribing information for the most up-to-date recommendations on dose, precautions, and contraindications, and determining the appropriate usage for the product. This is especially important in the case of drugs that are new or seldom used.

Production Credits
Publisher: Kevin Sullivan
Acquisitions Editor: Emily Ekle
Acquisitions Editor: Amy Sibley
Associate Editor: Patricia Donnelly
Editorial Assistant: Rachel Shuster
Senior Production Editor: Carolyn F. Rogers
Marketing Manager: Rebecca Wasley
V.P., Manufacturing and Inventory Control: Therese Connell
Composition: diacriTech
Cover Design: Kristin E. Parker
Cover Image: © Andrei Iancu/Dreamstime.com
Printing and Binding: Malloy, Inc.
Cover Printing: Malloy, Inc.

Library of Congress Cataloging-in-Publication Data
Shockney, Lillie, 1953-
    Becoming a breast cancer nurse navigator / Lillie D. Shockney.
        p. ; cm.
    Includes bibliographical references and index.
    ISBN 978-0-7637-8494-2 (pbk.)
    1. Breast–Cancer–Nursing. 2. Hospitals–Case management services. I. Title.
    [DNLM: 1. Breast Neoplasms–nursing. 2. Breast Neoplasms–psychology. 3. Continuity of Patient Care. 4. Health Services Accessibility–organization & administration. 5. Nurse's Role. 6. Oncologic Nursing–organization & administration. WY 156 S559b 2011]
    RC280.B8S4945 2011
    616.99'4490231–dc22
                                           2009048360
6048

Printed in the United States of America
13 12 11 10 09   10 9 8 7 6 5 4 3 2 1

Contents

Preface

Over the last few years there has been an increased interest in "patient navigation." This is the term that most healthcare professionals have come to recognize, even if they aren't exactly clear what the purpose of navigation is or who specifically is to be serving in the navigation role. To some degree this is understandable, because the term has been used somewhat loosely including its use in marketing campaigns that try to lure consumers to a specific institution because it offers "patient navigators." Though the advertisement or commercial on the radio may not explicitly state what the navigator does for the patient, to the ears of a consumer or someone who knows they are about to become a breast center patient, the wording of such a service sounds like the woman is definitely going to benefit from it. The advertisements may even go as far as to say she will need a navigator in order to successfully receive her care in a breast center environment. And perhaps it is true. Given the complexities of the healthcare system today, we all would probably benefit from having someone else navigate our care.

As health care has become more fragmented, managed care companies have increased their oversight and have chosen to contract certain medical services from different healthcare facilities, rather than making it easy for the patient and having it all contained in one facility. Such situations can require an organized and savvy person to figure out how to navigate on their own. This can be particularly difficult when dealing with a stressful diagnosis such as breast cancer. The patient may have her mammogram at one facility, her biopsy at another, see a breast surgeon at a third location, have her surgery at a hospital setting, chemotherapy in a medical oncology outpatient clinic environment, and radiation at yet another location, which may be closer to her home. To make sure that her care goes smoothly, her healthcare team members communicate with one another. For her diagnosis and treatment to happen in an efficient and effective way requires a management engineer to orchestrate. Add to this that some patients are without health insurance, have little or no access to care, and you have a patient set up for a poor outcome. She deserves good quality care like anyone else. She needs an advocate to help her, though. Such an advocate is a navigator.

This book focuses on the responsibilities of a navigator with a clinical background, most commonly a registered nurse. There are some institutions who have employed social workers or nurse practitioners to serve in the navigator role. And there are some healthcare facilities who have used lay people to some degree to serve in a navigator capacity. What you will learn from reading this book is the clinical navigation model, which is the most popular model. To navigate a patient through complex surgery and adjuvant treatment, the clinical navigation model works effectively, and its success in achieving desired goals is able to be measured.

You will learn about the importance of starting from scratch by learning what your patients currently experience in the absence of a navigator helping them. You will learn how to create measurable goals so that your performance can be measured. In an era when the economics of health care are in a crisis, everyone must justify their value within the healthcare system, including someone fulfilling the role of a breast cancer navigator. (When someone cannot explain what they do, why they do it, how they do it, and demonstrate its measurable benefit from a quality of care perspective and financial perspective, the outcome can be a pink slip.) Detailed information is provided within these pages to guide you in establishing baseline data, defining measures of performance, and tracking your success and failures (remembering that a lot can be learned from doing it wrong the first time. As Mark Twain once said, "Failure is the opportunity to begin again more intelligently.")

When you have finished developing and implementing your navigator program for your breast center, I hope you will take pride in what you have accomplished. Consider publishing your success, showcasing your work to such organizations as managed care organizations and the Joint Commission, providing your patients (and consumers who may become future patients in your community) information about your program by documenting it on your breast center Web site, and including stories in your quarterly newsletters mailed to consumers about your navigation program. Equally important, connect with other breast cancer navigators, and share your wisdom. There are thousands of breast centers in the United States. They are all different in some way and their organization structures vary, but all share a common goal—to provide quality care to their patients. You are now stepping forward to help improve the care patients receive in the breast center where you work. Welcome to the world of navigation!

Lillie D. Shockney, RN, BS, MAS

About the Author

Lillie D. Shockney, RN, BS, MAS

Administrative Director, Johns Hopkins Avon Foundation Breast Center

University Distinguished Service Associate Professor of Breast Cancer

Associate Professor of Surgery and Gynecology, Johns Hopkins University

Mrs. Shockney is a registered nurse with a BS in Health Care Administration from Saint Joseph's College and a master's in Administrative Science from Johns Hopkins University. She has worked at Johns Hopkins since 1983 and has served as the Administrative Director since 1997. As Administrative Director she is responsible for the quality-of-care programs; patient education programs; the survivor volunteer team; community outreach at the local, regional, and national levels; webmaster, and patient advocacy.

Mrs. Shockney has written 12 books and more than 200 articles on breast cancer and is a nationally recognized public speaker on the subject. She serves on the medical advisory board of several national breast cancer organizations and is the cofounder and vice president of a national nonprofit organization called "Mothers Supporting Daughters with Breast Cancer."

She is also the recipient of the Global Business Leadership award, numerous community service awards, was the recipient of the Outstanding Women of America Award, in 1997 was awarded the Distinguished Graduate for Lifetime Achievement Award, and in 1998 received the National Silver Medal Award from the National Consumer Health Information Center. In 1999 she was the recipient of the National Circle of Life Award and the American Cancer Society's Voice of Hope Award; in 2001, she was the recipient of the ACS Lane Adams Award for Excellence in Caring; in 2000, she was selected as an "Unsung Hero" for breast cancer by Pharmacia & Upjohn's 2001 calendar. She also received the 2001 Lane A. Adams Award for Excellence in Caring from the American Cancer Society. In addition, Mrs. Shockney has received the 2002 Faces of Breast Cancer, ACS, and the 2002 Oncology Nursing Society Award for Excellence in Breast Cancer Education awards. In 2003 she was the recipient of the Impact Award from the National Consortium of Breast Centers. She was also the recipient of the Komen Award from the Maryland Affiliate in 2003. In 2004 she was a finalist for the Lance Armstrong Foundation's Spirit of Survivorship award and was selected as one of the Top 100 Women in Maryland for her leadership and community service efforts. Mrs. Shockney was selected by the Komen Foundation, nationally, to receive the 2005 Professor of Survivorship Award. In 2006 she was the recipient of the Spirit of Friends Award from Food & Friends and the Avon Foundation, and also received the Patient of Courage Award from the American Plastic Surgery Society. Mrs. Shockney was the recipient of the 2007 Yoplait Breast Cancer Champion award. She received the 2009 ONS Excellence in Survivor Advocacy Award and, also in 2009, she received the Maryland Daily Record Healthcare Hero—Nursing Excellence Award.

In 2008, the Johns Hopkins Board of Trustees made a decision to appoint her to a chair as a University Distinguished Service Assistant Professor of Breast Cancer. This is the first time in the history of the institution that a hospital nurse has been appointed to a distinguished service designation.

She serves as "Ask an Expert" for several breast cancer Web sites including Yahoo.com and the Johns Hopkins Breast Center's Web site. She chairs the National Consortium of Breast Centers QI Task Force. Mrs. Shockney also holds a faculty appointment as Associate Professor in the Departments of Surgery and Gynecology within the Johns Hopkins University School of Medicine, and is an active clinical researcher with a focus on quality-of-life issues for survivors.

CHAPTER 1

STARTING WITH THE BASICS

This chapter starts with defining and describing the functions, roles, and expectations of a breast cancer patient navigator, then provides information about the history of this role (always good to know the background of how something came to be).

FUNCTIONS, ROLES, AND EXPECTATIONS

WHAT ARE THE FUNCTIONS OF A BREAST CENTER PATIENT NAVIGATOR?

A breast cancer patient navigator fulfills a critical role for many patients who are just learning they have been diagnosed with breast cancer. It is not unusual for a patient to say in retrospect that she felt like her navigator was her "lifeline," her "go-to person," "her support," or "the one with the answers and solutions." If you are embarking on becoming a navigator or have just been requested to fulfill this role within your breast center, congratulations! Your role is not just important—it is vital for the patients you will be helping in the future.

WHAT ARE THE ROLES OF A NAVIGATOR?

First it's best to define a bit more what is meant by the term *navigation*. This term is loosely used today and can mean a variety of different things. It is not unusual for the leadership in your breast center to have requested that patients "be navigated," but they themselves are not exactly clear what they are asking you to do. What is usually meant by "navigating a patient" is that someone helps the patient move smoothly through the system, receiving the standard of care delivered efficiently and in an effective manner. The following is a list of roles that patients believe a breast cancer navigator plays:

- Helping someone along a pathway to wellness following a diagnosis of breast cancer

- Scheduling tests and appointments for me

- Educating me about my treatment options and helping me figure out what happens next

- Psychological support during my treatment

- Helping me get through the maze of cancer care from surgery, chemo, and radiation, to survivorship

- Making sure I don't drop through the cracks along my treatment path

- Helping me with barriers that disrupt my treatment happening efficiently

- Finding financial resources to help me get my treatment paid because I lost my health insurance when I got laid off

- Helping me get a screening mammogram because I had been afraid to get one before

- Helping me get in to see a doctor when I found a lump in my breast

- Helping me find resources in my community that could assist me with child care and transportation so that I could keep my chemotherapy appointments and not miss any of them.

- Matching me up with a breast cancer survivor volunteer to talk with. This helped me emotionally as I took this long journey of breast cancer treatment. She had the same stage of disease and treatment that I had. She was all done though, and I couldn't wait to be like her. I would never have met her had it not been for my navigator.

- (from a husband) Helping me get linked with hospice and other agencies to help my wife and me, actually my whole family, prepare for losing Mary. She also helped us with our financial worries by connecting us with resources to help cover a lot of expenses I otherwise would have had to paid for out of pocket. Breast cancer treatment is expensive. It's even more expensive toward the end of life. Each day we had with her was a gift. I would have gone into great debt to have her here longer with us. Our navigator showed us ways to get support, including financially, so that we didn't have to go in debt.

- I don't know what it is, but I decided to go to the breast center because they advertised that they have a breast cancer patient navigator for newly diagnosed patients. That sounded good anyway. I don't think I ever met her though.

All of these statements made by patients are accurate regarding how an individual patient might define her experience with navigation (including the statement about hearing it as part of a marketing campaign but not experiencing it when she got her actual treatment). It is important that you have a clear understanding of how the breast center where you are working, most particularly the leadership of the center, define navigation and measure your performance before you even begin your orientation for this role.

WHAT ARE THE PATIENT'S EXPECTATIONS OF A NAVIGATOR?

Whether your patient heard an ad on the radio, read about patient navigation in literature she received from someone, or simply is applying her own knowledge of what she thinks of when she hears the word *navigation*, she probably has a preconceived idea, to some degree, about what she expects to be done for her and with her by you. Listed below are some common statements from patients describing what they believe the role of a patient navigator is:

- Guide her through a complex maze of appointments, procedures, tests, decision-making steps, and actual treatment of her breast cancer.

- Reduce her anxiety about treatment by empowering her with information and reducing obstacles of concern.

- Help her overcome any communication gaps that exist between the providers of her care and her and her family.

- Make the breast cancer treatment experience manageable, as she continues with her life.

- Remove barriers impeding her care and treatment.

WHAT MIGHT BE THE BREAST CENTER LEADERSHIP'S EXPECTATIONS OF YOU AS THEIR NAVIGATOR?

Not only is it important to know what your patient may be expecting of you but also what your boss expects as well. More details will be provided about this later in the book, as we look at ways to measure your success. Some common themes of expectations are listed below:

- Improve efficiency in delivery of care and treatment.

- Increase patient satisfaction.

- Reduce physician time in the clinic and on phone calls from patients.

- Ensure continuity of care and coordination of that care.

- Serve as quality control.

- Identify and eliminate barriers to care— systemically from an operations management perspective as well as individually for patients.

- Track data for quality measurement.

- Improve clinical quality and service.

See the importance of your role now? Sound like it is too hard to accomplish? It is not intended to be done in a vacuum alone. Remember that. You are one member of the breast center team. Collaboration is key. There are always bumps at first while you are still learning the best way to efficiently carry out your work. The next section discusses the history of patient navigation.

THE HISTORY OF PATIENT NAVIGATION

Is patient navigator a new role for healthcare professionals? Not exactly. Let's look at the history—if we don't know where we've been, we may not understand where we are now and where we may be heading in the future. In the late 1970s and early 1980s the government decided to implement major changes in how hospitals would be paid for providing inpatient care. Healthcare expenses had been recognized as being out of control even back then. A patient went to the hospital the day before her operation, spent the night, and stayed in for many days afterwards until she felt well enough to go home. For a woman having a mastectomy, the average length of stay was 7 days. This healthcare finance system was called prospective payment, and codes were assigned to each diagnosis and procedure. In turn, specific amounts of reimbursement were provided based on the diagnosis (including comorbidities) a patient had and the procedures she underwent. This amount of money and defined number of days allocated for the hospital stay were tied to a specific DRG (diagnosis-related group). When a patient exceeded the length of stay or maxed out the dollar limit dictated by her DRG, the hospital finance department knew it would not be receiving any additional money for the care they were providing this patient. There were some exceptions, such as specific complications or comorbid conditions that a patient might have that could bump her up to a higher-paying DRG, but the system was imperfect. If, however, the patient was discharged prior to her designated number of days or before the expenses associated with her care were spent, the hospital would make extra profit.

As a way to monitor this process, utilization review was conducted. Utilization review (UR) is a process for monitoring the use and delivery of services, especially one used by a managed care provider to control healthcare costs. There were "UR nurses" employed by insurance companies to retrospectively review medical records and determine if there had been inappropriate utilization of hospital or professional resources. Days of hospitalization that occurred on weekends when radiology services weren't available or an extra night in the hospital because the patient didn't have someone available to drive her home were closely scrutinized. Doctors and the hospital received "denial letters" from UR departments at managed care organizations. Organizations overseeing Medicare and Medicaid (called peer review organizations [PROs]) informed doctors and hospitals that certain days of care or tests that were performed on the patient during her hospitalization would not be covered. Such decisions were often hard to reverse. There were situations in which patients were prematurely discharged from hospitals because the patients had reached their DRG limit. In an attempt to anticipate which patient's records might result in the issuance of a denial letter, hospitals employed UR nurses as well to perform the same chart review task. These individuals would inform the finance department of potential risk of financial loss based on their medical record review. In some cases, the hospital UR department also sent letters to the doctors informing them of the same and requesting that they explain why care was delivered in a less than optimal manner. The reality of the situation was that the patient had gone home and the doctor was now busy taking care of new patients. His interest in explaining why the radiology department isn't open on weekends or why the patient requested to stay an extra day was the least of his current worries. What was more concerning were the situations in which patients were prematurely discharged resulting in poor care being provided.

In the late 1980s, changes were made to this way of monitoring care, and utilization management was introduced. Utilization management (UM) is the evaluation of the appropriateness, medical need, and efficiency of healthcare services, procedures, and facilities according to established criteria or guidelines and under the provisions of an applicable health benefits plan. Though the overarching goal, according to the government and managed care organizations, was to help ensure patients were provided cost-effective, high-quality, medically necessary care delivered in an efficient manner, the managed care organizations as well as the government (PROs) overseeing Medicare and Medical Assistance still had an adversarial relationship with doctors and hospitals. The mission was to avoid delays in treatment and delays in discharge from the hospital for inpatients receiving care, no matter what their disease or disorder was. Diagnosis-related groups (DRGs) were still the payment system. Insurance companies invested a great deal of money in performing, in a concurrent manner, reviews of medical records of hospitalized patients.

UM nurses monitored a patient's hospitalization to ensure each day was medically necessary, there were no barriers to treatment or barriers to her being discharged to home, and she had a good clinical outcome. Hospitals now employed their own UM nurses (many of whom were previously UR nurses) to review the medical record documentation each day during the patient's hospitalization and contact the doctor if there were any barriers to treatment or to her discharge that she identified. The most common problem was lack of documentation in the medical records by the doctor to justify the medical necessity for the patient to be in the hospital on a given day. Keep in mind too that up to this point whether it was the UR process or the UM process being followed, neither the review nurses working for the outside organization or the nurses doing chart review inside the hospital had any contact with the patient. There were also situations in which the hospital UM nurse was responsible to contact the insurance carrier's UM department each day and report on what specific care was being provided to the patient in order to justify her staying in the hospital "one more day." Quality of care was getting more attention now, however, and patient safety was starting to surface. PROs in particular were monitoring care from a quality perspective, raising flags when a complication would occur that was felt to be avoidable. Such instances could result in a team of doctors and nurses coming to the hospital and conducting focused reviews of specific patient populations. There was a war continuing between payers of care and the providers of care.

In the early 1990s this process evolved yet again. Case management was born. The definition and philosophy of case management was quite different than what had been conducted previously under the UR or UM program models. Based on the needs and values of the patient and in collaboration with all her healthcare providers, the case manager (again a role fulfilled by a nurse) linked patients with appropriate providers and resources through the continuum of health and human services and care settings, while ensuring that the care provided was safe, effective, patient centered, and delivered in an efficient manner. Finally, the patient was involved, and the nurse was involved with the patient. The role went from an adversarial one to one of collaboration. The case manager was considered a vital member of the healthcare team. The case manager had hands-on involvement with the patient, performing the following tasks:

1. Addressed barriers to care by ensuring that tests happened in a timely manner

2. Educated the patient about her disease and its treatment

3. Arranged consultations for planning the next phase of care

4. Ensured that the team members involved with delivering care were communicating with one another

5. Addressed psychosocial and financial issues that might impact care or delay it

6. Arranged home care if a patient needed additional medical care after discharge.

TABLE 1-1 § History of Patient Navigation

1970: Utilization review	Monitor use and delivery of services	Adversarial	Inpatient	Retrospective chart review
1980: Utilization management	Evaluate appropriateness, medical need, efficiency	Adversarial	Inpatient	Concurrent chart review
1990: Case management	Assess, plan, implement, coordinate, monitor, evaluate	Collaborative	Involved in patient care	Hands-on care
1990: Patient navigation	Identify, reduce barriers to access to care, diagnose, prescribe	Collaborative	Underserved patients	Community outreach
2000: Patient navigation	Identify, reduce barriers to access care, diagnose, prescribe	Clinical collaborative	Across continuum of care, hands-on	Hands-on care and coordination of care

A particular focus, initially, was on patients with medical disorders who needed to be managed in a less expensive healthcare environment—either nursing homes, rehab centers, or at home with nurses or aides. Finally the healthcare system was no longer just focusing on charts and dollars but was focusing on the patient. Granted, having the patient's hospitalization not exceed the DRG limit was important, but greater emphasis was placed on improving efficiency in the care delivery process, engaging the patient in her care, and carrying the management of her care over into the outpatient setting. There are even some who would say that case management and patient navigation are the same thing.

As time progressed and more and more care became outpatient based, which was somewhat better reimbursed and less expensive than inpatient hospitalization, the focus needed to change once again in how care was managed and monitored. As you're no doubt aware, when a patient is in an inpatient bed today that person is very sick. Though utilization management programs are still in operation, justifying medical necessity for the patient staying in the hospital is rarely an issue today. And though more and more care is delivered in a more appropriate healthcare setting, it remains expensive—that's why the government and managed care organizations are continuing to look at alternative ways of delivering and paying for health care.

During the time that utilization management was being established, attention was being paid to issues associated with access to care. Dr. Harold Freeman, who coined the term *patient navigation*,[1] brought to the attention of healthcare professionals some important information that once again changed how the delivery of healthcare services, especially those for cancer care, would be conducted. The central issue Freeman identified and championed was that patients face a variety of barriers to standard cancer prevention information, screening, diagnosis, treatment, and follow-up care that inhibit timely access to healthcare services. These barriers include fragmentation of health-care services; lack of health insurance or being underinsured; provider- and patient-related education barriers; communication barriers, particularly for patients whose first language is not English; inadequate transportation to medical appointments; and missed appointments due to travel, child care, or employment barriers. Freeman also pointed out that health disparities arise when the delivery system does not provide access to timely, standard cancer care to everyone who needs it.[1] This was particularly evident among racial and ethnic minorities, people of low socioeconomic status, residents of rural areas, and members of other underserved populations.

Working at Harlem Hospital, Freeman implemented patient navigation to address this health disparity issue. This greatly broadened the spectrum of care. Up until then, the focus had been on patients who were already familiar and "in" the healthcare model, who had insurance coverage of some kind, and were undergoing treatment for a disease or disorder that had already been diagnosed. With patient navigators, the focus would begin much sooner—with routine screening, in the case of breast centers, mammography screening. Navigators were responsible for educating the community about breast cancer and recruiting patients to come to the mammography facility for screening and, if needed, diagnostic evaluation.

The goal of patient navigation according to Freeman (and later adopted by the National Cancer Institute[2]) is to facilitate timely access to quality, standard cancer care in a culturally sensitive manner for all patients. Examples of navigation services include facilitating communication and information exchange for patients with a limited understanding of the English language; coordinating care among medical service providers; and arranging for financial support, transportation, or child care services. Navigators under this model could be community lay persons or healthcare professionals. Patient navigation was to span the period from cancer detection procedures (i.e., screening mammography) through cancer diagnostic tests, to completion of treatment. This, of course, wasn't just an issue isolated to Harlem Hospital. The Institute of Medicine (IOM) report, *Care without Coverage: Too Little Too Late*,[3] states that uninsured patients get about one half the health care of insured patients and consequently die sooner than insured patients, largely because of delayed diagnosis. Another IOM report, *Ensuring Quality Cancer Care*,[4] cites concerns about lapses in care that can lower the chances of receiving the standard of care and compromise the quality of life and survival of cancer patients.

With the transference of care from an inpatient setting to an outpatient setting, and managed care dictating where a patient can have their treatment, more and more of the burden of keeping the schedule straight, understanding the sequence of care and treatment that lies ahead, and figuring out how to go from step 1 to step 2, rests on the shoulders of the patient. Whether the patient has cultural barriers, financial barriers, or racial barriers, the healthcare system has become incredibly complex. For a woman newly diagnosed with cancer, figuring out what happens next, what to expect, and how to ensure she is getting appropriate care is overwhelming without help. Patients and their families are so scared and shocked by the diagnosis that navigating through decision making about treatment options as well as actually receiving the multimodality treatment in a reasonably smooth way is considered nearly impossible. In the early 2000s the patient navigator role was expanded to encompass all patients and not just those who fit a specific underserved definition. (A summary of the history of patient navigation is provided for you in chart form on page 11, Table 1-1.) This doesn't mean that it has only been in the last few years that breast cancer patients have had someone to help them along this journey. Technically, everyone involved in her care and treatment has always had some role in navigating the patient along the decision-making and treatment pathway, but this process was fragmented and had no way to assess its effectiveness. In the past, each healthcare provider has focused on his or her specific portion of care, not necessarily looking across the continuum of care. Offering designated patient navigators has become popular in the last few years and particularly so in breast centers. The patient diagnosed with breast cancer should have positive expectations of what such an individual can do for her.

A strong focus remains on addressing the needs of the underserved, recognizing that their need for patient navigation is the highest among all populations. The President's Cancer Panel (2001)[5] reported on barriers, including system barriers (fragmentation of care), financial barriers (lack of insurance or being underinsured), physical barriers (excessive distance from treatment facilities), information and education barriers (both provider and patient related), and the issues of culture and bias. Other barriers that were identified that must be overcome include insufficient culturally sensitive information and educational materials for cancer patients and their families; inadequate transportation assistance to get to medical appointments; missed appointments due to travel or childcare barriers; patients' fiscal inability to take time off from work for screening and wellness care; and failure of providers to obtain patients' medical test or laboratory results in a timely fashion. Cultural and language barriers usually affect members of underserved populations. The cumulative effect of these barriers is unequal delivery of cancer prevention services and delays in detection, diagnosis, and quality treatment of cancers. Many racial and ethnic minorities, people of low socioeconomic status, residents of rural areas, and other underserved populations facing such barriers give up out of frustration or misunderstanding and drop out of cancer care services.

Patient navigators in a breast center may function similarly to a case worker, helping to shepherd underserved women in for screening mammograms and education about breast cancer and breast health. This navigator may remain involved through the patient's diagnosis or treatment, or the navigator might transition the patient to another navigator whose focus is on the diagnosis portion or treatment portion of breast cancer care. Some institutions do both types of navigation—prediagnosis and postdiagnosis.

These functions are rarely done by the same person, with one being based in a community setting having a liaison role with the breast center, and the other being physically based at the breast center. There are also breast centers who have mammography technicians within their imaging facility who fulfill the role of navigator from the time the patient comes in for her screening mammogram to when the patient is being diagnosed by having a biopsy done in the imaging facility.

In April of 2008, C-Change, a national cancer coalition comprising key national leaders from the government, business, and nonprofit sectors, hosted an educational briefing for members of Congress at the US capital. The vision and mission of C-Change is to eliminate cancer as a public health problem as soon as possible by leveraging the expertise and resources of its members. The organization strives to accelerate cancer research, improve the timely access to the full continuum of quality cancer care services, and support state, tribe, and territory comprehensive cancer control efforts.[6] The Cancer Patient Navigation Act was discussed. At this historic meeting, cancer patient navigation was discussed at length as was its importance in ensuring that cancer patients receive coordinated and high-quality patient-focused care. Patient navigation was referred to as the individualized assistance offered to patients, families, and caregivers to help overcome healthcare system barriers and to facilitate timely access to quality medical and psychosocial care from prediagnosis through all the phases of the cancer experience. Navigators guide a patient through the physical, emotional, and financial challenges that come with a cancer diagnosis.[7]

The Cancer Navigation Act, signed into law in June 2005, proposed spending $25 million over 5 years for demonstration projects that provide navigator services to improve health outcomes. In FY 2009, C-Change and other cancer leaders asked Congress for the $25 million needed to fully fund the act.

REFERENCES

1. Harold P. Freeman Institute for Patient Navigation. Fact Sheet [Web page]. New York: The Institute, 2009. Available at: http://www.hpfreemanpni.org. Accessed November 5, 2009.

2. Patient Navigation Research Program, Center to Reduce Cancer Health Disparities, National Cancer Institute. PNRP Brochure. Rockville, MD: National Cancer Institute, 2009. Available at: http://crchd.cancer.gov/attachments/pnrp_brochure.pdf. Accessed November 5, 2009.

3. Institute of Medicine. Care without coverage: too little, too late. Washington: National Academy Press. Available at: http://www.iom.edu/en/Reports/2003/Care-Without-Coverage-Too-Little-Too-Late.aspx. Accessed November 5, 2009.

4. Institute of Medicine. Ensuring quality cancer care. Washington: National Academy Press. Available at: http://www.iom.edu/en/Reports/2003/Ensuring-Quality-Cancer-Care.aspx. Accessed November 5, 2009.

5. National Cancer Institute, Division of Extramural Activities. President's Cancer Panel Annual Report for

2000-2001 with Video. Available at: http://deainfo. nci.nih.gov/advisory/pcp/video-report.htm. Accessed November 5, 2009.

6. C-Change. About C-Change. Available at: http://www. c-changetogether.org/about_ndc/default.asp. Accessed November 5, 2009.

7. Bio-Medicine. Support for Patient Navigation Services to Help Cancer Patients. Available at: http://www.bio-medicine.org/medicine-news-1/Support-for-Patient-Navigation-Services-to-Help-Cancer-Patients-17607-1. Accessed November 5, 2009.

CHAPTER 2

GETTING STARTED IN YOUR NAVIGATION ROLE: WHERE TO BEGIN

KNOWLEDGE BASE NEEDED

Before you can really get underway with navigating a patient, it is expected that you have a relatively sound foundation of medical knowledge regarding breast health and breast cancer and its treatment. Use this list below as a check list. Mark those areas you feel particularly strong in and those you want to learn more about to feel confident in your scope of knowledge. Your knowledge base needs to include the following:

- Screening mammography processes and protocols

- Diagnostic evaluation processes and protocols

- Biopsy procedures

- Pathology biopsy results including prognostic factors and their meaning

- Surgical treatment options

- Reconstruction treatment options

- Pathology surgical results including prognostic factors and their meaning

- Chemotherapy and targeted biologic therapy protocols and options

- Clinical trials available at your institution

- Radiation therapy treatment options

- Hormonal therapy treatment options

- Genetics and high-risk evaluation

- Survivorship care needs

- Treatment for all stages of disease (0–4)

- Treatment considerations for locally advanced disease

- Treatment considerations for elderly patients

- Treatment considerations for metastatic disease

- End-of-life issues

References to help you increase your knowledge on specific aspects of diagnosis and treatment information are *Johns Hopkins Breast Cancer Handbook for Health Care Professionals*, *100 Questions & Answers About Advanced and Metastatic Breast Cancer*, the NCCN breast cancer treatment guidelines available online at www.nccn.org, and the book, *Navigating Breast Cancer: A Guide for the Newly Diagnosed.*

COMMON BARRIERS

In addition to your medical knowledge, you need to have an understanding of the potential reasons why a patient isn't able to successfully access care or receive the standard of cancer care treatment. Some of the more common barriers are listed below. You may add additional ones to this list as you begin your role of navigator and identify additional barriers that exist within your community or that affect specific patient populations in your region. Common barriers to diagnosis and treatment include:

- Financial and economic

- Language and cultural

- Communication

- Healthcare system

- Transportation

- Bias based on culture, race, or age

- Fear

ADDITIONAL KNOWLEDGE YOU WILL NEED TO PERFORM YOUR JOB WELL

- Be knowledgeable about the psychosocial issues patients and families face associated with breast cancer.

- Gain experience as a good patient educator with solid communication skills.

- Learn what resources are available locally and regionally to support your patients.

Additional information of this type can be found at www.cancer.gov, www.cancer.net, www.breastcancer.org, and www.cancer.org.

CHAPTER 3

A PREREQUISITE TO NAVIGATING A PATIENT

EXPERIENCE YOUR BREAST CENTER THROUGH THE EYES OF A PATIENT

Before you can become a navigator proficient in your work, you need to experience your breast center from the other side—as a patient. Not literally but figuratively. Travel the same journey your patient takes. Walk in her shoes (or in this case, wear her bra). Don't assume you know all the steps even if you've previously been working in your breast center. You will have a bird's eye view if you literally spend some time observing the process yourself, documenting what you see, and before long, the barriers to inefficiency and the communication gaps will be staring you in the face. If your role begins at the time the patient is diagnosed, begin at the point the patient is called back after having had a screening mammogram that warrants more diagnostic workup. Flowchart each step looking at the process from an operations management perspective. Put a time line to what you see. Remember to record the "who does what, when, where, how, and why." Be prepared to be surprised.

DOCUMENTING THE PATIENT FLOW PROCESS

The following pages contain various tools and resources to help you get started or to further enhance your success as a breast cancer nurse navigator. As mentioned previously, it is very hard to navigate someone without knowing the patient care flow process yourself. A key component of your job focuses on ensuring that patients are diagnosed and treated promptly. This means that you need to know how efficiently the current care delivery model in your breast center works and identify ways in which it can be improved.

Table 3-1 provides you a template for recording information about your patient flow process. The comments section allows you to record information that may help you to identify barriers that are prolonging a time lag between one step and the next step along the continuum of care. For example, you note that there is a long time lag between the patient's postoperative appointment with the surgeon and her appointment to next see a medical oncologist about systemic treatment. Investigating who is responsible for making that medical oncology appointment and when it is arranged can give you key information as to how to shorten that time lag. If medical oncology appointments aren't scheduled until after the patient sees her breast surgeon for her postoperative evaluation, then the time lag could be several weeks. If, however, the medical oncology consultation was scheduled proactively at the time that the surgery was arranged, then the time lag can be dramatically shortened.

There may be additional steps in the process that you want to include too, such as notifying the clinical trials office of a potential patient for a research study, referring the patient to be fitted for a wig, signing her up to join the breast cancer support group, and having additional imaging studies performed. This chart however is a starting point for you as you create your own patient flow time line that matches the processes of care that occur in your setting. Keep Table 3-1 in mind while you read the examples on the following pages showing how implementing a small change in the process can positively affect patient care.

Now that you've had an opportunity to give some thought to the patient flow process, let's take a look at what impact making just a small change in the care delivery process has on improving efficiency, effectiveness, and overall quality care.

Table 3-2 shows specific phases of care, measured in time, for you to see how establishing a baseline of information, implementing a change, and remeasuring the process of care results in an improvement that can be documented and best of all then implemented as the new standard of care delivery in your setting.

By making changes when the medical oncology appointment is scheduled, as shown in Table 3-2, the patient can start chemotherapy 2 weeks sooner.

Examine the scenario in Table 3-3.

TABLE 3-1 ⸹ Flow Chart Depicting the Current Patient Flow Process in Our Breast Center

Process Being Performed	Average # of Days to Next Step	Comments
Recruitment of patient to have screening mammogram		
Screening mammogram performed		
Screening mammogram read by radiologist		
Patient informed of abnormal results		
Patient scheduled for diagnostic mammogram/US		
Referring physician notified		
Patient scheduled for biopsy/educated re: procedure		
Biopsy performed in breast imaging setting		
Biopsy results available from pathology		
Referring physician informed of results being breast cancer		
Patient informed that pathology results are cancer		

Surgical consultation scheduled

Patient seen by a breast surgeon for consultation

MRI requested and ordered (if needed)

Results of MRI known and reviewed by surgeon

Plastic surgery consultation arranged (due to MRI findings)

Breast cancer surgery scheduled

Preop teaching scheduled

Preop tests and H&P scheduled

Surgery performed (mast with DIEP flap for example)

Pathology available from surgery

Receptors from pathology available from surgery

Oncotype DX ordered (if appropriate)

Patient returns for postop visit

continues

TABLE 3-1 ☜ Flow Chart Depicting the Current Patient Flow Process in Our Breast Center (continued)

Process Being Performed	Average # of Days to Next Step	Comments
Patient scheduled for medical oncology consultation (if needed)		
Patient seen by medical oncologist (if appropriate)		
Patient has staging workup (if needed)		
Results of staging workup available and reviewed by oncologist		
Patient receives teaching about chemotherapy regimen		
Patient begins chemotherapy regimen		
Cycle #1		
Cycle #2		
Cycle #3		
Cycle #4		
Patient scheduled for radiation oncology consultation (if needed)		
Patient seen by radiation oncologist (if needed)		

Education about radiation therapy conducted					
Simulation for radiation therapy scheduled					
Simulation for radiation performed					
Radiation therapy begins					
Radiation therapy completed					
Patient scheduled to see medical oncologist for hormonal therapy					
Patient begins hormonal therapy					
Patient monitored for adherence to hormonal therapy					
Patient scheduled for follow-up appts/ tests as needed					

TABLE 3-2 ↪ Comparison of Time Lag by Making a Change in the Scheduling Process for Postoperative Medical Oncology Appointments

Old Process	New Process
Patient scheduled for surgery 4/21/10	Patient scheduled for surgery 4/21/10
	Patient also scheduled for medical oncology appt 5/13/10
Surgery performed 4/30/10	Surgery performed 4/30/10
Pathology results available 5/5/10	Pathology results available 5/5/10
Patient seen for postop appt 5/6/10	Patient seen for postop appt 5/6/10
Patient scheduled for medical oncology appt 5/26/10	
Medical oncology consultation performed 5/26/10	Medical oncology consultation performed 5/13/10
Chemotherapy begins 6/2/10	Chemotherapy begins 5/18/10

For patients who meet specific criteria (early-stage breast cancer, hormone receptor positive, and HER2neu negative), there is an opportunity for the surgeons and medical oncologists to work as a team in determining who may benefit from having the Oncotype DX test performed. Rather than adding a delay in the process for getting these results back by having the test ordered after the patient is seen by the medical oncologist, the process can be speeded up by having the breast surgeon order the test based on criteria provided by medical oncology. In doing so, these results are available when the medical oncology consultation takes

TABLE 3-3 ⮎ Comparison of Time Lag by Changing When Oncotype DX Test is Ordered and by Whom

Old Process	New Process
Surgery performed 4/30/10	Surgery performed 4/30/10
Pathology results available 5/5/10	Pathology results available 5/5/10
Patient seen for postop appt 5/6/10	Patient seen for postop appt 5/6/10
	Oncotype DX test ordered by surgeon 5/6/10
Medical oncology consultation performed 5/26/10	Medical oncology consultation performed 5/15/10
	(Oncotype DX results available for appt)
Oncotype DX test ordered 5/26/10	
Results of Oncotype DX test available 6/5/10	
Consultation again with medical oncologist to discuss results 6/8/10	
Chemotherapy begins 6/13/10	Chemotherapy begins 5/20/10

place and decisions can be immediately made regarding whether the patient will or will not have chemotherapy. In the scenario depicted above, this speeded up the process by 4 weeks and saved the medical oncologist time by not having to meet with the patient a second time to review these results.

Examine the next opportunity for improving efficiency and expediting the patient's care and treatment in Table 3-4.

TABLE 3-4 ⌐ Utilizing Pathology Information from the Biopsy to Schedule Appointments in an Expeditious Way

Old Process	New Process
Bx results confirm inflammatory breast cancer 10/20/10	Bx results confirm inflammatory breast cancer 10/20/10
Patient scheduled for surgical consult 10/22/10	
Patient referred to medical oncology consult 10/22/10	Patient scheduled with medical oncologist 10/20/10
Patient seen by medical oncologist 10/26/10	Patient seen by medical oncologist 10/22/10
Staging workup performed 10/30/10	Staging workup performed 10/24/10
Neoadjuvant chemotherapy begins 11/5/10	Neoadjuvant chemotherapy begins 10/30/10

Though the time difference is "only a week" from the perspective of the patient, it can feel like a lifetime. By recognizing at the time the pathology results are available that the patient has inflammatory breast cancer, steps can be taken to fast track her to medical oncology to get underway with neoadjuvant chemotherapy. It can be quite distressing for a patient to see a surgeon first, be told that she is not operable, and needs systemic treatment before surgery can be considered. Her anxiety goes further up when told that she has to wait several days before seeing a medical oncologist. So in this scenario not only are you making sure the care is provided more efficiently, you are also addressing her psychological needs as well. The patient can see the breast surgeon during the week she begins her chemotherapy.

The surgeon can examine her and continue to see her during her systemic treatment with the goal of doing her mastectomy surgery when chemotherapy is completed.

SOFTWARE TO HELP YOU TRACK YOUR PATIENTS AND PRODUCE REPORTS

As you navigate more and more of your patients across the continuum of care, it will not take very long for you to begin feeling overwhelmed with keeping track of test results and the next steps you need to take to facilitate assessments, care, and treatment. You might begin using a Kardex system to record information. This can quickly become cumbersome and at times frustrating, especially if you are responsible for a large number of patients. One solution is to electronically capture the information via computer and let the software remind you what needs to happen next on any given day for your patients. Using navigation software can also ease the process when you need to be away and someone else is filling in for you.

Priority Consult Breast Care is a customizable and comprehensive breast patient navigation and clinical tracking computer program. Supporting both nurse and nonnurse patient navigators, the program assists breast center staff in directing and following a patient from initial screening or diagnostic imaging, to biopsy and pathology, through treatment and follow-up. Navigators responsible for patients at a particular stage in care benefit from a notification of a patient's status as well as a prompt when an action is scheduled to occur. This is done through the use of a sophisticated queuing and alert system that mirrors the breast care continuum. The queuing system enables breast center staff to view the status and next step of every active patient within the program. Information regarding a patient at a particular stage is gathered and stored within the Priority Consult Breast Care system. The information is used to create treatment summaries for members of the tumor board. Once a patient has been presented before the tumor board, a navigator can enter into the system the recommended treatment plan and use the information to help forecast, in an easy-to-understand visual form, what the patient can expect during the course of her treatment.

After a patient has been tracked through her treatment phase of care, a navigator can once again use the program to forecast a patient's next step—her survivorship plan. Custom survivorship planning documents are built into the software program and when generated, take into account the treatment a patient has received. Ongoing follow-up is managed through a queuing system that alerts breast center staff when it is time to complete scheduled follow-up. The software is also designed to report breast center clinical quality and operational efficiency indicators as laid out by such organizations as the National Quality Measures for Breast Centers. For more information regarding Priority Consult Breast Care, visit www.priorityconsult.com.

The next section is a case study that walks you through a patient's entire journey from the point of abnormal mammogram through the completion of her breast cancer treatment.

NAVIGATION EXAMPLE ACROSS THE CONTINUUM—A CASE STUDY

This case study uses the letters B, E, T, S, and Q to help define what the navigator should be identifying within any specific phase of a patient's care or treatment:

B — Define the *B*arriers to progressing the patient from one phase of care or treatment to another.

E — *E*ducate the patient.

T — *T*rack data to ensure quality control.

S — *S*chedule steps that must take place to navigate her to the next step.

Q — Identify ways to measure performance through the application of *Q*uality measurements.

Details are key here. As mentioned before, navigation cannot be done solely by one person. Knowing who is involved, what their responsibilities are, and how to communicate with them is critical to your success as a navigator.

While evaluating this process from an operations management perspective, pay attention to the following:

- Duplication of effort

- Delays in the delivery of care

- Whether the appropriate person is responsible for the appropriate task based on skill

- Knowledge, salary, and time allotted to accomplish it

Anticipate there being some changes in work flow as one of the outcomes of conducting this important analysis. What you want as an end result should be a well-oiled machine that functions smoothly, consistently, and reliably.

This case study serves as an example of what your role as navigator might be as you navigate a patient across the continuum:

> Screening mammogram (bi-rad 4) ▶ Diagnostic imaging ▶ Core biopsy

A 48-year-old patient came in for her routine screening mammogram on Thursday, April 2. She had no breast abnormalities to report. Her films were read the following day, and a spiculated mass was noted in the upper-outer quadrant of the left breast, measuring 1.3 cm. The breast imaging scheduler called the patient to inform her she needed additional imaging done. She was scheduled to return on Monday, April 6. The call was transferred to the navigator. The navigator did the following:

- Explained what a bi-rad 4 score on breast imaging means

- Inquired about medications the patient may be taking that might interfere with performing a biopsy the same day

- Educated the patient about diagnostic mammograms, breast ultrasound, spot films, and core biopsy procedure

- Reiterated time to arrive on Monday, and requested she bring a family member/friend to drive her home, given a biopsy may be performed the same day

- Inquired if there were any barriers that would prevent the patient from keeping her appointment for Monday (child care, copayments, fear, transportation, work requirements, etc.)

S   Patient needs to be scheduled for diagnostic mammogram, possibly ultrasound and core/stereo biopsy (factor in questions about blood thinners, local anesthetic).

B   Assess for barriers related to compliance with keeping appointment for diagnostic evaluation (getting off work, child care, copayments, lack of understanding of importance of keeping this appointment).

E   Educate patient about meaning of bi-rad score of 4.
Educate patient about purpose of additional imaging studies, such as spot films and ultrasound.
Educate patient about biopsy procedure.
Educate patient about how biopsy results will be provided to her.

T   Record the date of screening mammogram and date for diagnostic evaluation and biopsy.

Q   Time from screening to diagnostic mammogram.
Time from diagnostic imaging to biopsy.
Time from biopsy to pathology results known.

Time from pathology results available to when patient was informed about results.

Time from pathology known to patient to patient scheduled for consultation with a breast surgeon.

During these steps, the patient communicated with a breast imaging scheduler, a front-desk registrar, a radiologist, a mammography technician, and the navigator.

> Core biopsy ▶ Pathology results ▶ Patient notified ▶ Surgical consultation scheduled

Diagnostic evaluation and biopsy were performed on Monday, April 6. Biopsy was performed as a core biopsy in ultrasound. The patient was given postprocedure instructions by the mammography technician and told by the radiologist that someone will call her in a few days with the results. On Wednesday, April 8, the pathology results were available, and the patient was called by the radiologist to inform her that she had invasive ductal carcinoma. The navigator did the following:

- Informed the patient of her role in her care going forward, beginning with being present for her surgical consultation.

- Educated her about the medical terms in her pathology report from the biopsy procedure

- Determined if there were any barriers preventing the patient from coming to her surgical appointment, and bringing a family member or friend to accompany her

- Provided the patient an overview of what to expect during the surgical consultation

S Schedule patient for an appointment with a breast surgeon. Note patient is a biopsy-proven patient and should receive priority for being scheduled soon.
Schedule time with the navigator to coincide with surgical consultation.

B Identify any barriers patient may have regarding her ability to come in for her consultation.

E Educate patient about purpose of surgical consultation.
Instruct patient to bring family member with her.
Provide basic information about breast cancer diagnosis and treatment.
Provide information about the role of navigator in her care.

T Record date results being available from pathology.
Record date and time patient notified of results.

Q Time from core biopsy to pathology results available.
Time from results available to patient being notified of pathology results.
Time from patient notified of results to patient scheduled for surgical consultation.

During these steps, the patient communicated with a breast imaging radiologist, the mammography technician, the navigator, and the surgical appointment scheduler.

> Breast surgical consult ▶ MRI ▶ Plastic surgery consult ▶ Schedule for breast cancer surgery

The patient arrives for her appointment with the breast surgeon. During the consultation the navigator is present in the room for the clinical breast exam, review of the mammograms and ultrasounds, and the discussion about the surgical treatment options. The surgeon recommends that the patient see a plastic surgeon to review her reconstruction options if she decides to have a mastectomy instead of a lumpectomy. He also requests that she be scheduled for a breast MRI since her breast tissue is very dense so that multicentric disease can be ruled out and confirmation can be provided about how large the tumor appears to be. If lumpectomy is the option chosen, for which the surgeon feels she is a good candidate for, it will be done as a wire localization procedure. The navigator did the following:

- Reiterated the information provided by the breast surgeon

- Explained to the patient the surgical options, wire localization procedure, survival rate stats, and local recurrence stats for lumpectomy versus mastectomy options

- Explained to the patient what to expect during the plastic surgery consultation

- Showed the patient photographs of the various surgical options including lumpectomy, mastectomy, and mastectomy with various forms of reconstruction

- Assessed the patient's concerns related to intimacy and sexuality

- Provided the patient with an overview of radiation therapy treatment protocols and the necessity of radiation for women choosing lumpectomy

- Explained to the patient the breast MRI procedure, how it is done, and what information will be obtained from it that may affect decision making about surgical treatment

- Explained the sentinel node biopsy procedure and how axillary dissection is performed if the node is positive

- Assessed her for barriers that may affect the patient's decision making regarding her choice of surgical options (i.e., no transportation for coming daily for radiation therapy)

- Gave the patient educational information to take home with her as well as a list of resources pertinent to her for additional education and support

S Schedule patient for an appointment with a plastic surgeon in the breast center.
Schedule patient for a breast MRI (factoring in her menstrual history).

B Identify any barriers patient may have regarding coming in for her consultation or her MRI.

E Educate patient about survival stats and recurrence stats for lumpectomy with radiation versus mastectomy.

Educate patient about reconstruction options.

Educate patient about breast MRI procedure.

Educate patient about sentinel node biopsy.

T   Time from request for MRI to be scheduled to MRI being performed (exclude delay due to menstrual cycle).

Time from request for plastic surgery consultation to appointment taking place.

Q   Measure patient satisfaction with surgical consultation experience.

Length of time from consultation to patient being scheduled for breast cancer surgery.

Measure patient satisfaction with preoperative teaching.

The patient communicated with the breast surgeon and the navigator.

> Surgery procedures scheduled ▶ Preop tests and H&P arranged ▶ Preop teaching scheduled ▶ Patient goes to surgery

After the MRI and consultations are completed, the navigator confirmed there were no additional findings of concern on the MRI that could influence decision making about surgical options (i.e., no multicentric disease; tumor remained same measurement). The patient saw the plastic surgeon and discussed both implant and flap reconstruction options. The patient chose to do lumpectomy with sentinel node biopsy followed by radiation. The need for chemotherapy or hormonal therapy remain unknown for now. The OR scheduler arranged for preop tests, notified PCP of need for H&P to be done, and arranged the OR date and the preop teaching appointment. The patient had her H&P done by her PCP, along with blood work, chest X-ray, and EKG done the same day in his office on April 13. Her surgery was scheduled for April 15. The navigator did the following:

- Reviewed the results of the MRI and spoke with the surgeon to confirm that the patient remains a candidate for lumpectomy surgery if she chooses

- Reviewed the clinical note from the plastic surgeon to see the outcome of the consultation

- Contacted the patient to discuss her MRI results, her plastic surgeon consultation, and to discuss the patient's decision regarding breast surgical options

- Contacted the OR scheduler to facilitate scheduling of preop tests/procedures, H&P, as well as actual OR date

- Reviewed the PCP clinical notes to ensure patient was cleared for surgery

- Met with patient or communicated by phone to provide preop teaching information including what to expect throughout her surgery day, how she will feel afterward, wound care instructions, and the necessity to have someone accompany her since she will not be allowed to drive herself home that afternoon. The sentinel node procedure was reviewed in detail since she will be receiving a radioactive isotope injection in radiology before going to the operating room. The wire localization procedure was also explained in depth.

- Reviewed with patient the type of pathology information that will be learned from the surgery

- Reviewed with patient the time line for meeting with a medical oncologist and radiation oncologist and their roles in her adjuvant therapy planning process

- Followed up on preop test results to ensure there were no findings that affect surgery taking place as planned

S Preop tests, H&P, OR date, wire localization procedure preop, sentinel node injection preop. Postop appointment 1 week following surgery. Consultations postop with medical oncologist. Consultations postop with radiation oncologist.

B Assess for barriers related to preparing for surgery and immediate postop needs.

E Educate patient about preoperative instructions (NPO after midnight), wound care, sentinel node biopsy procedure, possible axillary node dissection teaching, wire localization procedure, 24 hours prior to surgery any drug administration instructions (related to her prescription and OTC drugs the patient takes on a regular basis).
Educate patient about what to expect at time of postop appointment with surgeon.
Educate patient about what to expect at time of medical and radiation oncology appointments.

T   Record the dates following appointments were scheduled: preop teaching; postop appointments—surgical, medical oncology, and radiation oncology. Record dates they actually occurred.

Q   No delays in surgical treatment due to failure to confirm preoperative tests completed and within normal limits; patient adequately prepared by participating in preop teaching; MRI imaging and mammography studies correlated with one another to ensure surgical recommendations do not require changing. Measure patient satisfaction with entire treatment process to date.

Patient communicated with the navigator, surgeon, OR scheduler, PCP, precare nurses, OR nurses, recovery room nurses, and anesthesiology.

> Discharged from ambulatory surgery recovery room
> ▶ Home care ▶ Postop surgical appointment

The patient's surgery is done. She underwent a wire localization lumpectomy with sentinel node biopsy. During the operation the sentinel node was sent to pathology for touch prep analysis and found to be positive for cancer. An axillary node dissection was performed on level I and II nodes and a drain placed. The patient was transferred to the recovery room. The navigator called the recovery room to get a status report on the patient. She was informed that the sentinel node was positive. The navigator provided the recovery room nurse with information about what preop teaching instructions the patient had had prior to going to surgery. The recovery room nurse reiterated drain care instructions with the patient and her husband. She was discharged to home with an appointment slip to return to see the surgeon in 6 days. The navigator called the patient the morning after surgery to see how she was feeling and how much drainage was coming from her axillary-placed Jackson Pratt drain. The patient returned for her postop appointment, had her drain removed by a nurse practitioner in the breast center, and was given her pathology results by the surgeon with the navigator present. Her incisions were healing well. Her tumor measured 1.4 cm of invasive ductal carcinoma. Margins were all clear for greater than 2 mm. ER was 90%; PR was 70%. HER2neu was negative. Grade 3. Ki67 was 70%. The sentinel node was positive for metastatic disease. No other nodes were positive. The total number of nodes removed was 12. The patient was told when she would be seeing the medical oncologist and radiation oncologist and the purpose of these appointments. In preparation for the medical oncology appointment, the navigator contacted the medical oncologist to obtain information about what tests would be desired to be performed prior to the consultation. The medical oncologist requested Oncotype DX, CAT scan, and bone scan be done along with a MUGA scan and blood work for the purpose of conducting a staging workup. The navigator did the following:

- Ensured the patient had clear instructions regarding her drain management and wound care at home

- Assessed her for psychosocial needs, with focus on new information that her nodes were positive

- Ensured she had her postop appointment for surgical visit next week

- Ensured she had contact information for medical emergencies/questions

- Reviewed the pathology report prior to the patient returning for postop visit to ensure it was available for time of visit, what the findings were, and its completeness for prognostic factors and staging information

- Joined the patient at the time of the postop visit with the surgeon to reiterate the findings and explain next treatment steps

- Reviewed the schedule to ensure the patient had information about date, time, and location for her medical oncology and radiation oncology appointments

- Explained what to expect at the oncology appointments

- Contacted medical oncologist to determine what staging workup tests would be desired for completion of staging information

- Explained to patient the purpose of these tests and how it relates to planning her treatment

- Arranged for these tests to be performed

S Order MUGA scan, bone scan, CAT scan, blood work, and Oncotype DX.

B   Assess for any barriers preventing patient from having tests and medical oncology as well as radiation oncology consultation.

E   Educate patient about her pathology results regarding stage II breast cancer with favorable prognostic factors.
Educate patient about the purpose of additional tests being requested by medical oncologist in preparation for appointment.

T   Record the dates of her medical oncology and radiation oncology appointments and record when they were actually completed.
Record the dates the tests that were ordered were to be done and the dates when the results were back (should be prior to medical oncology consultation).

Q   Completeness of pathology report including all prognostic factors:
Postop wound infection rate
Seroma rate
Reexcision rate
Breast conservation rate (excludes multicentric disease and/or stage III patients)

Patient communicated with the navigator, surgeon, recovery room nurses, and breast center NP.

> Staging workup tests ▶ Medical oncology consultation

The patient had her tests done and saw the medical oncologist the following week. Her scans were clear with no evidence of metastasis, and her MUGA scan was within normal limits. Her Oncotype DX score was 35. Based on the Oncotype DX score, age of the patient, and overall health, the medical oncologist recommended chemotherapy and hormonal therapy. The medical oncologist advised the use of specific chemotherapy drugs be given, spacing cycles 2 weeks apart, and felt she was a good candidate for the clinical trial X. The risks and benefits of treatment were reviewed in detail, and the patient agreed to participate in the clinical trial drug regimen. She received a total of 12 cycles of chemotherapy, combining a mixture of drugs over that period. She was followed by a medical oncology nurse practitioner closely for monitoring her blood levels, side effects, and temperature. The navigator spoke with the patient the day after her consultation to review with her the recommendations and address any questions she may have. The patient was concerned about side effects and her ability to work while receiving chemotherapy. The patient also didn't have money to purchase a wig and didn't want to start her treatment until she could afford to get a wig. The navigator provided her with free resources for obtaining a wig, reiterated the treatment regimen schedule, and the importance of keeping her appointments with the radiation oncologist next week as well as adherence to all her chemotherapy appointments. The navigator did the following:

- Ensured tests were performed prior to the patient seeing the medical oncologist

- Reviewed test results prior to medical oncology appointment

- Contacted patient one day after medical oncology appointment to review outcome of visit

- Assessed patient for possible clinical trials participation

- Provided information about chemotherapy schedules and monitoring during and between cycles

- Assessed patient for barriers that would prevent her from adhering to therapy recommendations

- Provided the patient with contact information to obtain a free wig from the American Cancer Society; checked with insurance company to see if they offer coverage for a "skull prosthesis"

- Ensured patient has transportation for chemotherapy appointments

- Reiterated purpose of chemotherapy and education information about the drugs and side effect management

- Confirmed patient has radiation oncology appointment for next week

- Assisted patient with marking her calendar with her chemotherapy treatments and home health needs

S Schedule chemotherapy treatment appointments every 2 weeks for 12 weeks.
Schedule appointments with medical oncologist and nurse practitioner alternating throughout treatment.

B Assess for barriers that affect ability of the patient to adhere to chemotherapy regimen.

T   Record and monitor patient's progress and compliance through chemotherapy treatment.

Q   Unplanned hospitalization during chemotherapy treatment.
Missed appointments for chemotherapy.
Adherence to NCCN treatment guidelines.

The patient communicated with the navigator, the medical oncologist, medical oncology NP, American Cancer Society office (for a free wig), and chemotherapy nurses.

Radiation consultation ▶ Chemotherapy treatment ▶ Radiation therapy treatment ▶ Hormonal therapy treatment

The patient met with the radiation oncologist the following week for consultation and discussion about radiation therapy that will begin after completion of her chemotherapy. She was educated about the purpose of radiation and how the therapy works, as well as the schedule for radiation. She completed her chemotherapy treatment with only having to delay one cycle of treatment by a week due to low blood counts. The navigator saw her during her treatment when she returned to see the surgeon 1 month and 3 months postop. The navigator also communicated with the patient by phone after each chemotherapy treatment and received reports from the chemotherapy nurse regarding her progress. She had one episode of nausea and vomiting that was not adequately controlled with the antiemetic drug she was given at the time of her initial treatment starting. She contacted the medical oncology doctor on call who prescribed for her a stronger antiemetic that relieved her of her symptoms. No hospitalization was required. She was educated about radiation therapy and given literature about this type of treatment. After a 2-week break postchemotherapy she met with the radiation oncologist again for treatment planning. Simulation was done at the time of the first visit, and 2 days later she began her daily radiation, Monday through Friday for 6 1/2 weeks. Other than fatigue, she did not have any concerning side effects. Upon completion of her radiation she returned to see her medical oncologist and received information about hormonal therapy and was given a prescription to start taking it for 5 years. She was given an appointment to see the medical oncologist again in 1 month. The navigator did the following:

- Educated the patient about chemotherapy, its side effects, ways to reduce side effects, and monitor her health.

- Instructed the patient about radiation therapy and the importance of adhering to the daily schedule.

- Taught the patient about hormonal therapy and the importance of adhering to the daily schedule.

- Assessed the patient for barriers that may affect her ability to stay on treatment regimens as prescribed.

- Provided the patient with information about long-term side effects of treatment including menopausal management caused by chemotherapy and hormonal therapy.

- Ensured the patient's appointments were scheduled at specific intervals following their departmental protocol for follow-up with the surgeon, medical oncologist, and radiation oncologist.

S   Appointments for chemotherapy administration. Appointments for blood work.
Appointments for follow-up with surgeon.
Appointments for ongoing monitoring by medical oncology team.
Appointments for ongoing monitoring by radiation oncologist.

B   Assess for barriers to treatment and adherence to schedule of treatment.

E   Educate patient about chemotherapy drugs, side effects, and overall treatment schedule.
Educate patient about radiation therapy regimen and overall treatment schedule.
Educate patient about hormonal therapy treatment and importance of adhering to taking medication daily and consistently.
Educate patient about potential side effects, with focus on bone health, menopausal management, and long-term side effects of chemotherapy and radiation therapy.

T   Record test results and when they were performed. Record patient's adherence to treatment schedule.

Q   Unplanned admission to hospital during chemotherapy.
Unplanned breaks in radiation therapy.

Compliance with adherence to hormonal therapy.
Adherence to NCCN treatment guidelines.
Measure patient satisfaction with treatment process to date.

Patient communicated with medical oncologist, radiation oncologist, navigator, NP, emergency on-call doctor, and American Cancer Society.

> Completion of adjuvant therapy ▶ Begin hormonal therapy ▶ Long-term survivorship monitoring

The patient has completed all her therapy with the exception of hormonal therapy. She is experiencing hot flashes and night sweats. She sees the medical oncologist 1 month after starting the medication. She complains of difficulty sleeping and feeling anxious since her chemotherapy and radiation ended. She is now seeing the surgeon every 6 months, medical oncology every 3–4 months, and radiation oncology every 6 months. The patient wants to have a CAT scan and bone scan repeated again and done at least annually due to fear of recurrence. The doctor told her that scans were no longer needed. The navigator did the following:

- Reiterated the importance of hormonal therapy for prevention of recurrence

- Discussed healthy lifestyle compliance to further reduce risk of recurrence

- Explained why scans are no longer routinely done posttreatment

- Recommended the patient attend an upcoming survivor retreat to help her with psychological issues she is experiencing, especially fear of recurrence

- Provided information and resources to help address menopausal symptoms

- Provided her information regarding survivor retreats and patient educational seminars

S   Long-term follow-up appointments with each oncology discipline.
Register patient for upcoming survivor retreat/education seminars for survivors.
Ensure patient is seen annually by her PCP for a physical exam.
Ensure patient is seen annually by her gynecologist for pelvic exam.
Ensure patient is scheduled for follow-up mammogram at specific intervals following institution's protocol for postradiation/surgical management of breast cancer.

B   Assess for barriers to adherence to hormonal therapy.
Assess for barriers to adherence for future appointments.

E   Educate patient about hormonal therapy, its purpose, side effects, and control of side effects.
Educate patient about long-term monitoring for recurrence or new onset of another cancer.
Educate patient about lifestyle changes that can further reduce risk of recurrence.

T   Ensure summary information about patient's entire treatment is documented and provided to her PCP and gynecologist.
Record compliance with follow-up appointments.

Record compliance with follow-up mammograms.
Record compliance with hormonal therapy as
prescribed.

Q   Measure psychological well-being at completion of
treatment and transition back to PCP.
Measure outcomes of participation in survivor
retreat.
Measure survival rate.

Patient communicated with navigator and majority of
her breast center team during this phase of care.

DEFINING WHEN NAVIGATION ENDS

This can be unclear in some cases. Patients may have developed a dependence on you that they don't want to lose. It is
important to establish guidelines; otherwise, you will find
your time occupied by the "worried well" who call you for
little things that take up time. As an example of this, should
the patient ask for an ultrasound when she gets her next
mammogram because her cancer was found with ultrasound?
Should she invest in brand-name vitamins instead of generic?

Work with your oncology team to determine the appropriate
time to transition her back to her PCP and gynecologist. For
women with early-stage breast cancer, their follow-up care
with the oncology team may be just a year or two whereas for
someone with stage III breast cancer, her long-term follow
up may be 5–6 years (provided she continues throughout this
time period to have no evidence of recurrence of disease).

NAVIGATING PATIENTS WITH METASTATIC DISEASE

What if your patient isn't going to be a long-term survivor? Though 85% of women diagnosed will be long-term

survivors and the mortality rate has been inching down over the last few years, this disease will still take the lives of 41,000 women and men in the United States in 2010. However, more women diagnosed with stage IV breast cancer are surviving longer and living with this disease as a chronic disease than ever before. With improvements in treatments, women can live several years to possibly a decade or more in some cases, always receiving some type of treatment to control the cancer where it has spread. The role of the navigator may be quite different from center to center. In some cases, a social worker may be assuming much of the responsibility. In other cases it may be the medical oncology nurse practitioner. Ensuring the patient has resources for support, information about hospice care services when appropriate, psychosocial support, and financial resources, are key.

MAKE SURE YOUR NAVIGATION ROLE IS CLEAR

You will still encounter people who, when you say you are a breast cancer patient navigator, look confused or simply tell you that they don't understand what you do. To help head off such confusion, particularly among other staff you are directly working with in the breast center, make sure your job description is clear regarding your roles and responsibilities. Defining your scope of practice is important for many reasons:

- It more clearly defines your responsibilities from that of others.

- It provides information from which performance measures can be developed and used

- It clarifies your role from that of the oncology nurse (at the bedside or in the clinic setting), the appointment scheduler, social worker, and even the clinical trials research nurse.

Saying you are a nurse navigator doesn't tell someone any specifics. If a nurse said that she is an oncology nurse and works in the chemotherapy administration area you could pretty much decipher what her roles and responsibilities are. Saying that you are a breast cancer patient navigator doesn't provide that same clarity.

Again, let's look at an example. You may be responsible to make sure the patient is scheduled postoperatively for her medical oncology appointment to discuss chemotherapy treatment. The appointment scheduler does the actual scheduling, however, based on the information you provide her; the clinical trials nurse assesses the patient's clinical information to see if she is a candidate for a specific clinical trial; the social worker may be involved in helping get the patient on medical assistance to cover the expenses of the treatment; and the oncology nurse is educating the patient about the specific chemotherapy drugs that will be used and administering these drugs following a specific schedule.

It is important for you to record specifically what you do, how you do it, when it is done, where it happens, and why.

Here's an example of a breast surgical consultation:

- Who—Navigator
- What—Arrange for patients surgical consultation appointments

- Where—In the surgical clinic of the breast center

- When—As soon as the biopsy results confirm a diagnosis of breast cancer

- How—By calling the appointment scheduler to procure an appointment and then calling the patient to inform her of the date and educating her about what to expect at the time of this consultation with a breast surgeon

- Why—To expedite the patient in getting evaluated and underway with a treatment plan; to provide the patient a point of contact to address her psychological needs and begin the education process overall about her treatment; and to provide her with a touchstone

MODELS OF PATIENT NAVIGATION

When developing a patient navigator program within your breast center, it is important to look at the organizational structure and determine what model will work best to address your patients' needs as well as what will be performed in an efficient and effective manner. The two current groupings for linking the navigator with the patient are:

- Matching navigator by tumor site (in this case, breast cancer)—a more clinically oriented approach

- Matching navigator by designated point of entry into the system—a more logistically driven method

There are variations within each given grouping. In 2008, the Oncology Round Table, based on surveys and interviews of breast centers that are part of their membership, outlined various methods that are used within these models. The six models listed below provide an overview of the most common variations within these two approaches. Dedicating patient navigators to a high-volume, low-acuity tumor site, such as breast cancer, remains the most common approach, as this allows for higher patient loads per navigator. Alternately, some designate a navigator to focus on high-acuity complex patients who have the greatest need for services, such as those patients diagnosed with pancreatic cancer or head and neck cancer. Additionally, underserved breast cancer patients may also fall into such a category owing to issues associated with noncompliance, literacy, lack of healthcare coverage, and other financial and culturally sensitive needs.

Over time the traditional navigation model has evolved to include a broad range of roles all aimed at expanding access to care and improving the patient experience. Many navigators today are responsible for organizing and coordinating the multidisciplinary case conferences (which are sometimes referred to as tumor board meetings) and multiple clinics in the center. Also, to increase the number of underserved women coming to the breast center for screening mammograms and potentially diagnostic needs and breast cancer treatment, time is also dedicated to performing various outreach efforts in local communities by raising awareness and creating a process to make it easier to bring patients in for their routine mammography screening and clinical breast exam.

Tables 3-5 and 3-6 show in chart format the two models referenced above.

TABLE 3-5 〜 Group I: Navigators Designated by Tumor Site

	Model I: High-Volume, Low-Acuity Tumor Sites	Model II: Low-Volume, High-Acuity Tumor Sites	Model III: All Tumor Sites
Description	Navigator assigned to high-volume, low-acuity tumor sites	Navigator assigned to low-volume, high-acuity tumor site(s)	Navigator assigned to provide coverage for all tumor sites
Rationale	Most commonly selected model as high-patient volumes tend to warrant assignment of a full-time equivalent	Patients with high levels of acuity tend to have a greater need for navigation services	Provides access to all cancer patients

Recognizing universal need, benefit across tumor sites |
| Site | Breast cancer | Head and neck cancers

GI cancers | All cancer types |
| Caveat | Although acuity is low, ensure volumes are appropriate given navigator staffing | Level of frequency, intensity of navigation services likely to be high; consider role modifications | Varying patient volumes across groups may necessitate assigning several tumor sites per navigator |

Source: Adapted from Oncology Roundtable. *Elevating the Patient Experience: Building Successful Patient Navigation, Multidisciplinary Care, and Survivorship Programs.* Washington, DC: The Advisory Board Company; 2008.

TABLE 3-6 ∫ Group II: Navigators Designated by Patient Entry Point

	Model IV: Multidisciplinary Clinic	Model V: Physician Based	Model VI: Community Based
Description	Navigator assigned to tumor site-specific conference/clinic	Navigator assigned to work with several physicians	Navigator assigned to subset of population experiencing disparities in care
Rationale	Ensures timely case presentations, follow-up coordination	Provides assistance when need identified; opportunity to increase physician efficiency	Identifies, addresses gaps in access, use of cancer service(s)
Site	Patient identified by referral, clinic visit	Patient identified by lead oncology physician	Patient identified in community by navigator
Caveat	Navigator clinic preparation, follow-up workload likely to vary by tumor site	Physician may request services beyond scope of navigator role Difficult to manage workload given physician variance	Funding commonly an issue; consider grant, foundation funding opportunities

Source: Adapted from Oncology Roundtable. *Elevating the Patient Experience: Building Successful Patient Navigation, Multidisciplinary Care, and Survivorship Programs.* Washington, DC: The Advisory Board Company; 2008.

Model I: High-volume, low-acuity tumor sites—
              This is most commonly used for new
              navigation programs just getting started.
              Maintaining a high and consistently
              stable volume helps too in justifying the
              presence of a full-time navigator. Usually
              the nurse navigator begins intervention
              at the diagnostic evaluation process or
              at the time the breast biopsy in breast
              imaging is confirmed to be breast cancer.

Model II: Low-volume, high-acuity tumor sites—
              This model is more commonly used
              in a clinical environment where the
              patients are going to need a great deal of
              time and resources to coordinate their
              care. Pancreatic cancer, lung cancer,
              head and neck cancer, and gynecologic
              oncology cancer patients are examples of
              these patient populations. Much of the
              care is provided in an inpatient hospital
              setting. Though volumes of patients are
              lower, they are known for being resource
              intensive.

Model III: All tumor sites—The cancer center
              determines that all patients are likely to
              benefit from patient navigation services
              to some degree. Individual navigator
              roles and responsibilities may actually
              vary, based on the type of cancer the
              patients have. This can be a more
              complicated model if the navigators are

reporting to one leader overseeing patient navigation versus reporting to a clinician leader within the specific tumor site.

Model IV: Multidisciplinary patient navigator— Such an individual would be responsible for providing logistical support to multidisciplinary conferences and clinics ensuring all the patient materials needed for case presentation are available and prepared for presentation, and the patient is informed of the outcome of the team's discussion. She assumes responsibility for time management of the conference itself. She also is responsible for coordinating follow-up care for the patient based on the decisions and recommendations made by the team.

Model V: Patient navigators provide coverage via assigned physicians—This enables the navigator to intervene when physicians identify specific patient needs. In additional to performing the standard navigation role of identifying and eliminating barriers to care, this model also aims at increasing physician's efficient use of time by intervening at the actual moment when needed. To work well, standardization of this role is needed due to variation in the use of the navigator by various doctors.

Model VI: Patient navigator to address regional disparities—This really is where navigation was born (see the history of navigation section of this book). The navigator may be working in several different sites within a geographic region where patients are known to have significant gaps and barriers in accessing cancer services and care. This requires partnerships with other organizations. It also requires the navigator to develop site-specific programs focusing on promoting awareness, prevention, and screening. She may transfer a patient to a navigator at the breast center once the patient has been diagnosed with breast cancer.

Whatever model you choose to adopt, be sensitive to the fact that this takes time to create. Selecting a model is just one of the steps you will take when considering how to develop and implement a navigation program that works to address your patients' needs and supports the mission and scope of practice of your breast center. Plan carefully. It can be easy for a navigator to become over-whelmed early on because of high volume and the failure of having resources in place to address the barriers as you identify them and work to eliminate them. Working efficiently is key. It will not always be possible to meet with a patient face to face to carry out a certain task on their behalf. You may be communicating with them via phone or e-mail.

You may even decide during the development process to implement two different models and compare the results in order to determine what model will serve your patients and organization best. This doesn't happen overnight. The final outcome however should be that your patients see a smooth delivery of care that to them looks seamless. This is like putting on a major event. To those who attend it, it needs to look like it was easy to orchestrate and pull off. For those of you who have planned large events, you know how time consuming the details and planning process can be before the big night actually happens. Once you've held the event though and done a debriefing afterwards of what worked well, what didn't and how you want to improve it for next year, you soon find that during the fifth or sixth annual breast cancer gala event, the time needed to do the planning and coordination is much less than it was the first 2 years. The same applies to implementing a structure and process for patient navigation. Look at the current process, identify your barriers, select solutions (resources) to eliminate the barriers, measure how well it is working, and revisit the process again. Your patients will be the benefactors of your hard work behind the scenes, and as you adjust the process you will find more time to work on additional ways to make their patient experience the best it can be.

Though this book is geared toward nurse navigators, there are some breast centers who have opted to have other professionals as well as lay persons fulfilling some level of navigation for their patients. Who is doing the navigation and what their educational background and skills are directly affects what level of navigation they can perform.

The following sections examine six different categories of navigator role based on the individual's training and education:

VOLUNTEER NAVIGATOR

During hard economic times, more and more institutions are revisiting the roles they have volunteers fulfilling and expanding those responsibilities to be more directly involved with direct patient contact. A volunteer is able to connect patients to educational information resources and community resources. There is of course no direct financial cost to the breast center, except for minimal HR requirements such as TB testing, policy and procedure training for hazardous waste, and other universal training requirements of personnel who have physical contact with a patient. Someone to supervise the volunteer is also required, as well as training this individual in carrying out her tasks. Determining how to measure her effectiveness in doing these tasks must also be developed. You may have a volunteer(s) working with you to assist you with clerical functions that otherwise you would be doing yourself which is not a wise use of nursing resources. Volunteers however are, well, volunteers. They don't have to show up for work. Turnover can be a problem in some environments. It's harder to discipline someone who isn't doing a good job but wants to give of their personal time.

AMERICAN CANCER SOCIETY NAVIGATOR

This individual is dually trained by the breast center and by the American Cancer Society (ACS). They are to serve specific roles and use standard information, including resources available through the ACS network. The cost is usually relatively low as the ACS is providing this individual through a grant to the institution. The breast center may be picking up part of her salary and benefits, but the ACS navigator is a shared resource with the ACS. The downside is that they may be restricted in what they can and cannot do since the ACS has implemented a specific model across the country and has it uniformly delivered.

LAY BREAST CANCER SURVIVOR

This woman is able to connect patients with information and resources they need. It costs less than a clinical professional. This individual can be used to assist you in your work. The downside is that the individual lacks medical knowledge beyond her own experience. Even if she is a healthcare professional of some type, if she is fulfilling the role as a volunteer or lay person, then she is not at liberty to provide medical information or advice. Her value may be in providing psychological support.

SOCIAL WORKER

Her background does allow her to assess the patient for barriers and address her psychosocial needs as well as provide initial counseling. This level of healthcare professional is less expensive than an RN or APN while still having some level of clinical knowledge. She is usually very familiar with community resources and how to use them. She is restricted in her level of medical knowledge and her ability to address treatment and symptom concerns the patient may have.

NURSE

This is the most common model today. The background of a registered nurse (RN) provides patients with medically knowledgeable resources, and she is trained to conduct a nursing assessment. She is able to play a larger role in the patient's care because she is a clinician. She is also able to refer patients to support services as needed. Though she may lack familiarity with community resources, she can learn this information relatively quickly by interacting with the oncology social worker team as well as making visits to these resources in the community herself. This model is a more costly model than social worker or nonclinical individuals but remains the most popular one adopted by breast centers today. Fifty-five percent of navigators currently working for cancer centers are RNs.

ADVANCED PRACTICE NURSE

The advanced practice nurse's (APN's) background tends to bring more credibility to the navigator role from a physician's perspective. There is also the potential to be able to bill for navigator services within the nursing model of care. The APN is able to play a larger role, even beyond that of the RN if needed. Once she has learned what support services are available within the institution and local community, the APN can refer patients. This is the most costly model, and it can be difficult to justify the higher cost above an RN level unless the breast center implements a way to bill for the APN's services. Of navigators currently working in cancer centers, 205 are APNs.

CHAPTER 4

MEASURING YOUR IMPACT: HOW TO MEASURE THE BENEFITS OF THE NAVIGATOR PROGRAM WITHIN YOUR BREAST CENTER

The leaders of your breast center want to ensure the time and money they have invested in developing and implementing your navigator role provides the intended outcomes for patients and for the breast center as a whole. It is wonderful to have a patient tell you personally how helpful you have been in navigating them through such a life-altering experience as breast cancer diagnosis and treatment. Being able to demonstrate your value to leadership is also critically important, especially in hard economic times. Table 5-1 provides additional examples of ways to measure your performance as well as clarify your roles and responsibilities by isolating them from the responsibilities of others who work hand in hand with delivering patient care.

In times of cost containment in the healthcare arena, being able to justify a specific program, particularly if it is new and not a billable service, is paramount to the program continuing. The same applies to a navigation program. It is necessary to demonstrate its value to the overall patient care delivery system, as well as demonstrate that providing a coordinated navigation service enhances patient care, patient satisfaction, and results in more patients choosing to come to your breast center in the future. The following are some questions commonly asked when evaluating the success of a navigation program:

- What is the effect of the patient navigator assisting patients in coordinating services, from the point of a suspicious cancer finding through noncancer resolution or cancer treatment? Include overcoming such access barriers as financial, lack of information, and healthcare system barriers.

- To what extent does the type or degree of service result in reduction and/or elimination of patient-access barriers, thereby providing more timely access to quality standard cancer care for all patients?

- To what extent does demographic matching of patient and navigator (e.g., race, ethnicity, gender) or fluency in primary language of the patient affect standard of care adherence and perceived satisfaction with the healthcare system?

- How effective, in terms of cost and meeting the goals of the navigation program as set forth by the breast center leadership, is a patient navigator in providing patient support and assistance to eliminate patient access barriers and improve timely delivery of quality, standard cancer care?

The expectation is that navigated patients will (1) receive timelier, definitive diagnosis following screening and abnormal findings; (2) receive timelier treatments following a positive diagnosis of cancer; (3) improve their satisfaction with the healthcare system experience; and (4) result in more patients receiving appropriate treatment in keeping with NCCN treatment guidelines.

There have been a variety of models of navigation developed across the country, with the support of research grants from organizations such as the National Cancer Institute, Komen for the Cure, the Avon Foundation, the American Cancer Society, and other financial resources. Questions still being answered relate to what is the ideal navigation model. The real answer is that the model needs to be specific for the healthcare environment and patient population it is designed to serve. As an example, it may be important to have patient navigators who are laypeople working in the community who can conduct outreach and recruit African American women to come for screening mammograms. Studies thus far show the importance of such a "recruiter" (i.e., patient navigator) also being African American and living in the community she serves.

Studies have been launched in a variety of settings to scientifically measure how well various strategies fulfill the role of patient navigation. The questions being asked by the National Cancer Institute, who is one funder of navigation programs, include questions such as those listed above as well as the following:

- Which patient navigation strategies are most effective? Those of an indigenous nonprofessional (cancer survivor, community layperson) or those of a professional healthcare provider (nurse, social worker, or other allied healthcare professional)? Volunteer navigator or paid navigator?

- Does the primary location (community-based organization, primary care screening/diagnosis clinic/center, or hospital center) of the patient navigator affect the success of the navigation?

- Does the patient navigator assisting patients in coordinating care among multiple physicians affect standard of care adherence and perceived satisfaction with the healthcare system?

- Does a patient navigator assisting patients through the cancer care continuum increase patients' and their families' identification and use of a usual source of care, for both cancer follow-up and other medical conditions?

To demonstrate success with some of these specific thought-provoking questions, you need to ensure that your breast center has in place the resources to provide the services needed. You need to document the methodologies and techniques for overcoming barriers (e.g., utilizing a primary language other than English) to timely access to cancer diagnosis and treatment services. Your breast center needs to show an adequate breast cancer screening rate. These rates will ensure that a sufficient sample (based on power analysis of patients with abnormal findings) are referred to the patient navigator.

Don't make assumptions about what is needed to be accomplished through the development and implementation of a navigation program. Begin with the basics. This means performing a needs assessment. The next steps include selecting and training patient navigator(s), developing and implementing how patients are tracked, conducting a rigorous evaluation at specific intervals, and disseminating the findings to leadership and any organization that is a source of funding.

Start with collecting and recording baseline historical data and make plans for a continuous comparison group through the study period. It is important to factor in history effects, system biases, community activities that may affect changes in cancer disparities (e.g., other organization's efforts to increase cancer screening rates) and other confounding factors.

Your needs assessment will help to determine the most frequent patient-access barriers and identify methods and techniques to overcome these access barriers in a timely, efficient manner. You might even decide to try eliminating these barriers using several different methods and compare the methods to see which works best.

You and the breast center faculty will want to establish rapport with primary care and other cancer care providers and nursing staff in your community who you anticipate working with. If you are targeting a specific neighborhood to increase mammography screening rates, reach out to the primary care physicians (PCPs) in that area, as well as the community centers, churches, and other local organizations to make them aware of your intended efforts and goals of the program. If your focus is on increasing screening rates, you also need to know the community screening rates and number of abnormal findings currently in the cancer care continuum. Some data you need comes from Medicare information or Medicaid data base.

It is terrific when you see the community working together. You can keep records of the number of patient referrals you receive for screening mammography appointments from Dr. X (the PCP in the targeted community). He is making the referrals when he sees patients for common colds and flu. This is teamwork at its best—bringing community outreach, patient navigation, and community providers together for a common goal: to increase compliance with annual mammography screening. Purchasing cab vouchers and engaging the local cab service to pick a patient up for her screening mammogram and return at a designated time to take her back home brings in other community resources that result in an increase in access to care.

Do not think that you will remember each implementation step you have done. Record them as you implement them. Revisit your list often to see where you have been and where you are going. Make incremental changes. Rome was not built in a weekend, neither will your navigation program, not a successful one in any case.

When you are just beginning your navigation role, it can seem difficult and quite complex to figure out what measurements you want to undertake first. It is to your advantage however to start from the onset of the implementation of your position to measure the impact your work has on contributing to improving the delivery of patient care. So consider starting with a list of overarching goals you want to accomplish and demonstrate your direct contribution as a nurse navigator has on breast health and breast cancer patient care. Here are areas of focus to consider when developing ways to specifically measure the value of a formal navigation program at your institution:

- Improved coordination of high-quality care:
  - Demonstrate that patients are not falling through the cracks as they are transitioned from one discipline (surgical oncology) to another (medical oncology and radiation oncology).
  - Demonstrate that there are not delays in providing this coordination.
- Enhanced access to services for all patients:
  - Measure the frequency of support services being used by patients (matching with a survivor volunteer for support; ACS road to recovery; wig closet; cancer counseling center).
  - Increase the number of underserved patients having screening mammograms.
- Removal of barriers to care:
  - Track these barriers by type and record how each barrier was overcome:
    - Financial and economic
    - Language and cultural
    - Communication
    - Healthcare system
    - Transportation
    - Bias based on culture, race, or age
    - Fear

- More efficient delivery of care by measuring the time delays from one point to the next (turnaround times for results; appointment requested and appointment taking place)

- Improved outcomes
  - Compliance with providing care that meets National Comprehensive Cancer Network (NCCN) treatment guidelines
  - Survival rates
  - Stages of disease at time of diagnosis
  - Adherence to treatment

- Improved sharing of resources, such as demonstrating avoidance of rework and duplication of administrative tasks or patient education

- Enhanced relationships with the community:
  - Use of community resources
  - Recruitment of patients for screening mammograms from the community through awareness efforts and events

- Increased patient satisfaction, including specific satisfaction survey questions directed at navigation program

- Increased referrals of new patients to the system:
  - Include the source of the referrals (patient, referring physician)
  - Referring physician satisfaction

Here is a list of qualitative and quantitative measures to consider when providing a monthly report to your breast center leadership (and grant funding source organization):

- Number of patients referred

- Stage at time of diagnosis

- Appointments kept and missed and reasons

- Number of patients accepting navigation

- Number of current dependents in patient's family

- Reasons for accepting or not accepting navigation

- Baseline knowledge of cancer treatment options

- Education and information materials provided to patient and family members

- Patient demographics (e.g., race/ethnicity, age, socioeconomic status, primary language)

- Patient access barriers and time to resolve each barrier, including issues addressed in resolving access

- Distance of patient's home from diagnosis and treatment facilities

- Recommended diagnostic procedures and adherence to schedule

- Patient's primary mode of transportation to diagnosis and treatment facilities

- Recommended treatment procedures and adherence to treatment protocol

- Other nonaccess-specific navigation services requested or provided

At a minimum, include the following outcome measures:

- Changes in time from abnormal finding to diagnosis or other resolution

- Positive diagnosis to treatment implementation

- Improvements in satisfaction with breast center care experience

Cost-effective measurement outcomes are important and include:

- Labor cost of the navigator

- Cost of training the navigator

- Time navigator spends on various activities: contacting patient, coordinating patient records with providers, overcoming various types of access barriers such as arranging transportation, community education about navigation process, and similar patient navigation activities

- Patient follow-up surveys to measure patient and family changes in knowledge of breast cancer prevention and early detection (following community education events or screening mammogram)

- Patient satisfaction with her experience at the breast center including her time spent with the navigator

As you become more seasoned in your role you will be able to advance your measurement process further to include process evaluation measures that can include what characteristics are important to the patient navigation process. Examples include the following:

- What services are critical to provide to the patient—for example, only overcoming cancer care access barriers or also emotional, psychological, and referral support and access for medical treatment?

- What training and support is critical to the patient navigator—cancer prevention control, hospital procedures and administration, medical knowledge, and/or emotional and psychological support to minimize burnout?

- How many patients can a patient navigator effectively assist simultaneously?

- Do other program linkages and partnerships or other agencies have an impact on the success of the patient navigation intervention strategies?

Feeling overwhelmed? Don't be. Chapter 5 will provide you examples of exactly how all of this can be done.

Case Study Example of How a Navigation Program May Be Developed, Implemented, and Its Success Measured

L ooking at how specific components of a navigation program were implemented elsewhere can be helpful in getting you launched in doing the same at your breast center. Though there are many more details behind this descriptive information, a work plan is provided as a way to give you a framework for creating your own development and implementation program.

NEEDS ASSESSMENT

The first step before developing and implementing a navigation program is to determine if there is a true need for one and what specifically is needed. Don't assume anything. What you personally think is a problem may not be. For example, you assume that women in the community are not getting mammograms because they are fearful of the results. You invest money in creating literature about the value of mammography and importance of early detection and distribute the literature through churches, grocery stores, and hair salons. But you notice no increase in the number of screening mammograms being performed at your facility. You later learn that community residents are more than willing to come in for screening but lack insurance coverage. They didn't know you had a free screening program they can use. Oops. Take the time to do surveys, review statistics, conduct interviews, and gather unbiased information. It is best to make hypotheses and then validate them through the needs assessment process.

GATHERING AND ANALYZING DATA

To start your needs assessment you will probably need the following information. The types of statistics listed here are not all from one institution and are merely intended to provide some structure to the workflow process you will need to create for yourself:

1. Data from external resources includes screening mammography statistics such as what Medicare and Medicaid can provide regarding the rate of compliance with annual screening mammography, and demographic data (e.g., geographic, economic status, age group) about the population you are striving to serve.

   a. This information shows you that about 40% of women who are candidates for screening mammography are actually getting their annual mammogram.

2. The American Cancer Society can provide you with statistics by zip code of the volume of breast cancer

patients diagnosed as well as statistics on the stages of the disease. Your tumor registry at your hospital also has this type of data.

a. From this information you learn that more than 70% of women diagnosed in your targeted zip code are diagnosed with locally advanced disease.

b. The incidence of diagnosis is less than it is for other communities too, implying that women are going undiagnosed.

3. Internal data within your breast center including the volume of screening mammograms performed, no-show rate in mammography for screening and diagnostic imaging, catchment area for your breast center geographically, stage of diagnosis and number of patients diagnosed with breast cancer, patient satisfaction data, payer data, compliance information on your own patients regarding adherence to NCCN treatment guidelines

a. This data informs you also that patients from the targeted area are diagnosed with stage III or IV breast cancer 70% of the time.

b. Despite having the resources for providing chemotherapy and radiation therapy, 40% of patients needing this treatment do not receive it.

c. The no-show rate for screening mammography is 22%.

d. The no-show rate for diagnostic imaging is 45%.

e. 28% of patients in "d" are lost to follow-up.

f. 21% of patients in "a" and "b" are lost to follow-up.

g. The number of patients coming in for screening mammography from the targeted catchment area is low.

4. Conduct interviews with community doctors (primary care physicians, gynecologists), community leaders, and breast center faculty and staff to learn their thoughts on where the needs are as well as what their specific needs are as healthcare professionals.

a. Primary care physicians and gynecologists tell you that they are happy to refer their patients in for screening mammograms but know their patients have difficulty taking time off from work or getting child care, which has resulted in their own patients also missing doctor's visits with them as well.

b. Community leaders tell you that they want to hold health fairs in the city several times a year to improve wellness and healthy lifestyle habits by offering free blood pressure checks, cholesterol screening, smoking cessation programs, and diabetes screening. They are also interested in working with the hospital to raise awareness about breast cancer, prostate cancer, cervical cancer, and HIV.

c. The breast center faculty and staff tell you about how difficult it is, once a patient comes in for a screening mammogram, to subsequently contact the patient and convince them to return for diagnostic imaging when abnormalities are found.

d. Your oncologists talk about their frustration in taking a great deal of time trying to explain a treatment plan to a patient newly diagnosed who comes alone and seems to not understand the importance of compliance and adhering to the prescribed treatment plan.

e. The breast center nurses tell you that they triage a lot of phone calls from patients who are confused about what the next steps are in their breast cancer treatment plans and want to review it again with them, but the breast center nurse wasn't present with the patient when the consultation with the doctor took place.

f. Local clergy tell you that breast cancer stirs up great anxiety among their congregation since they have witnessed many African American women get diagnosed with metastatic disease, and therefore congregation members assume if you get diagnosed you are destined to die.

g. Mammography schedulers tell you of their frustrations in not being able to reach a patient when calling to have them return for a diagnostic mammogram. Their reasons were that there was usually no phone number to call, a bad address in the system, or noncompliance in the patient showing up.

5. Conduct surveys with consumers in the community.

   a. Consumers enlighten you to a list of myths that women have about breast cancer and its treatment:

       i. Mammograms cause breast cancer.

       ii. If you get breast cancer you will definitely die so don't put yourself through treatment for nothing.

       iii. Mammograms are expensive.

       iv. Being diagnosed with breast cancer when it is small doesn't make a difference in the fact that you will still die from it.

       v. If you don't have insurance, you can't get treatment.

       vi. Treatment (chemotherapy) can cause you to die, unrelated to having breast cancer.

       vii. There is no way to prevent breast cancer.

       viii. If you don't have it in your family, then you won't get it either.

       ix. Surgical treatment is always mastectomy.

       x. Radiation causes lung cancer.

       xi. If a local resident of the urban community goes to the hospital, they will be experimented on with breast cancer drugs.

6. Collate your results to identify what opportunities you want to address by creating a working list.

   a. Increase the number and percentage of women having screening mammography from the defined targeted geographic region.

      i. Current no-show rate is 22%.

      ii. 40% of women who are candidates for having annual screening mammograms are currently having screening mammograms.

   b. Increase the number and percentage of women having diagnostic mammograms.

      i. Current no-show rate is 45%.

      ii. 28% are lost to follow-up.

   c. Partner with the community health education/outreach programs to provide educational information to consumers about breast cancer and breast health—instilling the facts, undoing the myths, and ensuring that the local community is aware of the free screening mammography services available for women age 40 and older.

   d. Increase the number and percentage of patients having breast cancer treatment that meets the NCCN treatment guidelines.

      i. Currently 40% of patients are not receiving appropriate treatment.

e. Increase the number and percentage of patients being diagnosed with early-stage breast cancer; decrease the number and percentage of women diagnosed with late-stage breast cancer.

    i. Currently 70% of women are diagnosed with locally advanced disease.

f. Develop a working relationship with local PCPs to facilitate their patients in getting screened as well as getting diagnostic mammograms.

    i. No baseline data available beyond qualitative interview information confirming this to be a problem.

g. Decrease the volume of calls coming to the clinical nurses in the breast center by patients in need of clarification of their treatment plan.

    i. Data tracked for a 1-month period showed 26 phone calls that took approximately 310 minutes of nursing time to address.

h. Decrease the amount of clinic time the faculty spend reiterating the treatment options and recommendations for breast cancer treatment.

    i. Data from a 1-month period showed that on average the doctors are spending 50 minutes with the patient during the new patient appointment consultation.

i. Reduce the patient's fear about breast cancer treatment.

  i. Surveys conducted with the community showed that 70% of the time patients believe if you get the disease you are destined to die from it.

  ii. Surveys also showed that clinical trials are being confused with guinea pig experimental testing and is feared by consumers 35% of the time.

  iii. Survey data showed that due to lack of understanding about the diagnosis and treatment, patients are opting to not have treatment.

   1. 65% believed that they can't get breast cancer if it doesn't run in their family.

   2. 50% believed there was no way to prevent breast cancer.

   3. 35% believed that without insurance, screening or treatment is not possible.

   4. 28% believed that radiation treatment causes lung cancer.

   5. 68% believed that the only surgical option for treatment is mastectomy.

   6. 34% believed that mammograms cause breast cancer.

   7. 62% didn't know that free screening mammograms are available.

8. 35% of those without health insurance coverage didn't know that they might qualify for Medical Assistance insurance coverage or qualify for the state grant.

CREATING A PRIORITY LIST

Now that you know where your starting points are for measuring, you can choose to tackle each one or initially limit your navigation plan to priority issues as you begin improving access to care and ensure appropriate treatment takes place. It may not be realistic to try to address the entire needs list at once. Select a few to start with that you anticipate being manageable for you and your team. If you have an executive committee of your breast center, this is the perfect group to whom to present your list. They can assist with prioritizing it as well as inform you of their expectations from the perspective of a time frame for reporting back your progress. You in turn need to speak up and inform them of what resources you need their assistance with obtaining in order for these improvements in the delivery of patient care to be accomplished. Small successes early on can reap great rewards later by serving as a catalyst for further improvements in your breast center.

EXAMPLES FROM JOHNS HOPKINS

The next step is to pull together your breast center team to strategize how these problems (opportunities for improvement) might be addressed. Share the information you gathered from your needs assessment with your team and start developing your plan.

The following are some specific steps taken by Johns Hopkins to improve patient care through effective navigation and team work:

1. Addressing issues associated with *poor compliance with returning for diagnostic mammograms*, you might decide to change the way you schedule them. At Johns Hopkins we decided to eliminate the need for call backs completed. When a woman comes in from the community for a screening mammogram, her record is flagged. Her screening mammogram is read in real time while she is there. If an abnormality is found it is pursued immediately by doing the necessary diagnostic evaluation, and if warranted, a biopsy as well. To accomplish this:

   a. Changes were made in the way records were flagged for such appointments.

   b. Breast imaging radiologist's workflow was altered to accommodate real-time reading of screening mammograms.

   c. The workflow process for performing the screening mammogram by the mammography technician was changed to accommodate her need to have the radiologist read the mammogram immediately while the patient remained in the changing room, still gowned.

   d. The schedule was assessed and data captured regarding how frequently a screening mammogram on this patient population converts into a diagnostic mammogram. Open slots were created into the schedule in advance to accommodate a specific number of anticipated add-ons to the schedule.

e. The schedule was assessed and data captured regarding how frequently a diagnostic mammogram on this patient population results in the need for a biopsy.

f. Special hours were created for performing screening mammograms on the underserved population to make it easier for them to be compliant.

g. The (community) breast center patient navigator arranged for transportation for patients and facilitated child care.

h. An advanced practice nurse met with each patient while there for a mammogram and performed a clinical breast exam as well as taught the patient how to perform a breast self-exam. Additionally the nurse reviewed the patient's medical and personal history to determine if she had any risk factors predisposing her to developing breast cancer.

i. Patients undergoing a biopsy had a survivor volunteer in the breast center to provide emotional support during the procedure. The survivor volunteer also stayed in touch with the patient after the biopsy results were known. For those with a positive biopsy, the survivor volunteer remained in touch with the patient throughout her treatment experience for emotional support.

- Johns Hopkins outcome for this intervention:

  ○ No show rate went from 28% to 11%

  ○ Time and money was saved on (unproductive) phone calls requesting the patient to return

  ○ Elimination of postcards and letters notifying the patient of an abnormality that warranted return for diagnostic evaluation

  ○ Elimination of scheduling patients for biopsies after diagnostic evaluation

  ○ Patient satisfaction was high with the introduction of a survivor volunteer for support

  ○ Patient satisfaction was high with the introduction of a clinical breast exam by a nurse practitioner

  ○ Patients' knowledge of breast cancer and its treatment was improved

- A note of interest regarding this operations management change—the decision was made early on that we would not only implement these changes for underserved patients, but for all of our patients. These standards of practice have become our standard of care for all women coming to our breast center, including the reading of a screening mammogram in real time.

2. Increase compliance with the patient coming for her surgical consultation once diagnosed with breast cancer. Reduce time spent by the physician during the consultation in explaining the details of the breast cancer treatment plan recommended for the patient. Also decrease the time spent by NPs addressing calls coming from patients after their consultation was completed.

   a. A relationship was fostered early on between the breast cancer nurse navigator and the patient at the time of her biopsy by having the radiologist make the navigator aware of the patient being there and her biopsy status.

   b. A relationship was also fostered by the survivor volunteer who held the patient's hand during the biopsy procedure.

   c. Efficiency and compliance was improved by having the breast center new patient appointment scheduler provide information via mail or electronically to patients about what to expect at the time of their first consultation with the breast surgeon.

      i. Appointments for patients with a diagnosis of breast cancer were provided within 72 hours of their knowing their diagnosis. Patients received their biopsy results within 24 hours of having the biopsy performed. In some cases the patient was seen the same day the biopsy was performed when it was noted that the cancer was locally advanced.

d. A breast cancer nurse navigator who has an oncology nursing background and is also a two-time breast cancer survivor (there are two such individuals) meets with the patient at the time of the consultation and remained in the room afterwards to reiterate the plan of care and address questions. The doctor's time was reduced by enabling him or her to present the information once, have the navigator remain behind to reiterate the plan and address questions, then have the surgeon return for a few final moments to address any remaining questions that could not be answered by the navigator herself.

e. Rather than having the patient receive a phone call some time later to arrange for her surgery date, the time invested by each of the physician's secretaries previously doing this task was reallocated to one person who became the OR scheduler. The patient was taken by the navigator to the OR scheduler in the breast center and the surgery date and all preoperative tests were arranged prior to the patient leaving.

f. The Red Devils, a community nonprofit organization in Maryland that provides support services to breast cancer patients, were engaged to assist the breast center with providing transportation for appointments, cleaning services for the patient's home, food for the patient and her family, and prescription coverage for medications such as hormonal therapy.

g. Patients were provided preoperative teaching to learn about their surgical care in advance.

h. Patients were also given the opportunity to be matched to a survivor volunteer based on the patient's age, stage of disease, race, and anticipated treatment plan. This individual served as an extension of the nurse navigator in providing emotional support to the patient.

i. A nurse working closely with the surgeon as well as the nurse navigator stays in close touch with the patient throughout her surgical treatment and recovery.

j. The navigator is responsible to ensure that appropriate postop appointments are scheduled including the patient's 1-week postop appointment with the surgeon (at which time the navigator also sees the patient) and appointments with the medical oncologist and radiation oncologist.

k. Specific literature is provided to the patient as part of her educational process. The book *Navigating Breast Cancer: A Guide for Newly Diagnosed* is provided to all breast cancer patients along with specific educational materials that are tailored to her treatment plan (e.g., wire localization procedure, axillary node dissection, drain management, reconstruction, mastectomy, lumpectomy, and/or sentinel node biopsy).

- This navigation program component has been highly successful with patients appreciating the patient-focused aspect of care being provided. Patient satisfaction survey results reflect the success of the program. Physician's time spent reiterating information was dramatically reduced. Compliance with keeping their surgery appointment for their operation to be performed was nearly 100%.

- Additionally statistics are kept regarding our utilization of Red Devil services. The two nurse navigators are able to generate a facility fee for the time spent with the patient performing patient education, psychological support, and coordination of care for those functions that take place while the patient is physically on the premises of the breast center.

3. Undo the myths and instill the facts about breast cancer and its treatment by raising awareness within the community.

   a. A breast cancer awareness program was developed called Breastivals. This program, which was born on the Johns Hopkins University's Homewood Campus, was designed to provide a fun way for young women (and men) to learn about breast health and breast cancer with the goal being to teach young people how lifestyle choices can influence risk, the warning signs of a breast health problem, how to perform a breast self-exam, and a breast center hotline number to call was offered should any of them having any questions or concerns about their own breast health. Breast cancer organizations are invited to participate and are given a booth to display their literature and organization's offerings. The students visited each booth, answered a flash card question about breast health or breast cancer (multiple choice and true and false), and after visiting all of the booths and getting their Breastival card stamped for having visited each booth, they were then rewarded with "booby prizes." By making it fun and engaging, students attended and learned. (See details of the outcomes at www. hopkinsbreastcenter.org/artemis; search for Breastival.) As an outcome of the success of this program, we began holding mini Breastivals at shopping malls, church bazaars, health fairs, and other venues. At these locations, consumers were asked to answer three flash card questions to be rewarded with (booby) prizes. Magnets, pens, flashlights, antibacterial hand soap, pill containers, and other rewards are provided. On college campuses food is a good way to draw the crowd to your door. Only those students who visited every booth and turned in a completed Breastival card were able to get food tickets. Consumers attending then placed their completed Breastival card with name and contact information into a (grand DD cup) door prize box for a chance to win gift certificates provided by the local stores in their community.

b. Implement a training program for laypersons to become certified as breast health educators (Certification for Breast Health Educators program). This 3-hour program, developed by myself, has become endorsed by the American Cancer Society. It enables a woman in her local community to learn the basics of breast cancer diagnosis and treatment, the facts about breast cancer and breast health, the warning signs of a breast health problem, the value of mammography and clinical breast exam, and how to get information about free screening in her community. The training program is free and held three times a year. The participant makes a commitment, by attending and learning, to then conduct at least two educational programs in her local community using either a 30-minute or 60-minute PowerPoint presentation provided at the end of the training. She is responsible to keep track of the number of women reached with this education. All medical questions a consumer may have by attending a local education program are directed to me, with the certified breast health educator providing her with my direct contact information.

Since the inception of the program in 2001, more than 140 Breastivals have been held across the country on college campuses. Hopkins continues to hold our Breastival on our college campus, and we track the number of Breastival programs we hold in local communities each year. This information includes the number of women attending, flash card questions they have trouble answering correctly, questions consumers ask us regarding their own breast health or a myth they have heard, and keeping track of women needing follow-up contact for appointments in our breast center. (For more information on how to hold a Breastival in your community, contact me at shockli@jhmi.edu. Breastival resource and planning kits are available for $99.)

Since the inception of the Certification for Breast Health Educators program in 1998, more than 500 women have been certified, many of them breast cancer survivors. The American Cancer Society maintains the statistics regarding the number of programs conducted, their locations, and how many women were reached. (For more information about this program, contact Jessica Bernstein at the Mid-Atlantic office of the American Cancer Society at 410-931-6850.)

Now you have examples to relate to as you begin your needs assessment and creation of an action plan. As you begin more advanced navigation and measurement of the success of the navigation program, you will want to continue to identify ways to quantitatively measure the program's benefits to your patients and community at large. Take a look on pubmed.com for published work on navigation programs that have been implemented elsewhere and how they have been successful in achieving goals that you might share with them.

Need more examples? Table 5-1 provides you additional examples of specific measures and how you might go about collecting patient-specific information to demonstrate your value as a breast center patient navigator.

TABLE 5-1 ⟿ Examples of Potential Measurements of Performance*

If you are responsible for being the first individual to provide support to the patient and facilitate their experience within the breast center, then you may want to consider measuring the *retention rate of your patients*:

- # of patients receiving breast surgical appointments for breast cancer surgery consultations: 52

- # of patients who stayed with the breast center and had their breast cancer surgery here: 51

- Retention rate 51/52 = 98%

One patient chose to go to a competing breast center. She was unhappy with the time frame offered for when the surgery would be performed (3-week wait).

If you are responsible for *expediting the patient to be seen by a breast surgeon* and are intervening at that step, then you may want to consider measuring the time lag from pathology results known to patient to when she is seen by a breast surgeon.

- Average length of time from confirmation of diagnosis to time seen by surgeon: 3.2 days

If you have a role in ensuring patients are receiving appropriate treatment in *keeping with NCCN treatment guidelines* you may consider measuring information related *to radiation oncology therapy* for patients having had lumpectomy surgery:

- # of patients who had lumpectomy surgery: 40

- # of patients referred for radiation therapy: 39

- % of patients referred: 98%

One patient was not referred. She is elderly, suffers from dementia and congestive heart failure, and lives in a nursing home. Wide margins were obtained, and the case presented to the tumor board to confirm that radiation therapy would not be necessary for this specific patient.

continues

TABLE 5-1 ⌐ Examples of Potential Measurements of
Performance* (*continued*)

Second opinions are a common reason a newly diagnosed breast
cancer patient will seek an appointment at a breast center. She has
been diagnosed elsewhere and already seen by a breast surgeon
and is coming for either confirmation of the recommendations
already received or perhaps is interested in determining where
she actually wants her surgery to take place and by whom. In
some breast centers, one of the roles of the navigator is to
educate the patient about the various services and programs
available to her at the center that she may want to consider receiving
as part of her care. One-on-one support from a survivor volunteer,
one-on-one patient education, state of the art reconstruction, and
of course, navigation would be examples of those services. If your
responsibility is to encourage a second-opinion patient to stay at
your breast center for her treatment, and the patient does, this is
again valuable information to capture and report as part of her
performance evaluation.

- # of second-opinion patients seen by breast surgeons: 14

- # of second-opinion patients who chose to have their
  surgery here: 10

- Capture rate: 10/14 = 71%

- # of second opinion patients seen by a medical oncologist: 10

- # of second opinion patients who chose to have their
  chemotherapy here: 8

- Capture rate: 8/10 = 80%

- # of second opinion patients seen by a radiation oncologist: 12

- # of second opinion patients who chose to have their radiation
  treatment here: 8

- Capture rate: 8/12 = 75%

  ○ If you are able to obtain financial reports, consider submitting
    a list of the patient's history numbers to your financial
    statistician so that revenue can be also part of your reporting
    information. Showing specifically how much revenue

continues

TABLE 5-1 ↪ Examples of Potential Measurements of Performance* (*continued*)

converting patients to choosing your breast center for their care can easily demonstrate the value of your position and potentially aid you in gaining additional resources when needed. (money talks)

Consider developing a *patient satisfaction* tool to be completed by the patient after the completion of her treatment. It should include specific questions regarding her navigation experience and be tied to your role and responsibilities. Measures could include the following questions (on a scale of 1–5):

- Ease of reaching the nurse navigator to ask questions and get support: 4.2

- Speed with which the patient's appointment was scheduled with the breast surgeon: 4.3

Remember too that anytime you are working with a team to improve a specific process, formally document the baseline measurement, steps taken to improve the situation, and the new measurement results achieved. When various accreditation organizations such as the American College of Surgeons or the Joint Commission come to conduct their triannual surveys, this type of information can be used as an example of *performance improvement*.

*These are examples reflecting a month of detailed information.

To help you further, check out the appendix that contains information of value to you as a navigator as well as organizations and educational resources for your patients. You are also welcome to review our data over time regarding our breast center performance, across the continuum of care. It is available at www.hopkinsbreastcenter.org. There you will find our 82-question patient satisfaction survey results that span more than a decade of tracking feedback from our breast cancer patients. You are also welcome to use this survey tool.

CONCLUSION

So let's recap for a moment. I started out with the basics to provide you with a foundation of knowledge beginning with understanding the importance of defining your functions and roles, and expectations of your leadership in your job. Next I provided you a summary of the history of patient navigation dating back to the 1970s with retrospective utilization review processes.

Then I moved you forward into understanding the importance of where your roles and responsibilities are to begin (and end), and the clinical and psychosocial knowledge you will need in order to do your job well. This was followed by providing you with information about the most common types of barriers your patients may present with that are key to address so that she receives her care in an efficient and reliable manner.

Next was information about the importance of viewing the breast health/breast cancer experience in your institution through the eyes of your patients, and to make no assumptions about how you think things work within your own doors. Then you learned how to document the patient flow process and identify delays in the process as well as potential duplication of effort that need to be addressed from an operations management perspective. An overview of navigation software was next discussed with the intent to ease the burden of manually tracking your workload. I then provided you with a case study so that you can "experience" navigation and see your role across the care continuum for a breast cancer patient.

I then provided you information about various models of navigation including the categories of navigators who are in such positions in various breast center and cancer centers across the country.

This was followed by a dedicated chapter on how to measure your impact as a nurse navigator—the benefit to patients from a quality of care perspective and the benefit to the breast center from a financial and clinical operations perspective.

Another case study was then provided to walk you through how to develop and implement a patient navigation program in your institution. This included gathering analysis data, doing a needs assessment, and other measurements. I also provided you with actual examples from the Johns Hopkins Breast Center's work we have conducted in that area.

The appendices are important for you to review, too, so don't close the book yet! Once you have more experience in your role, you should seriously consider getting certified as a navigator as well (see the NCBC certification program in Appendix A).

I know you will do a great job, now that you have the tools to do this important work. Though you will experience other barriers, some perhaps even political, that may arise periodically, remember to stay focused on the patient's needs. You (and I) are here for our patients. Let's help them have an experience that is the least physically and emotionally traumatic we can provide for them as they take their journey with the diagnosis and treatment of their breast cancer.

RESOURCES FOR YOU AND YOUR PATIENTS

BOOKS

FOR YOUR PATIENTS

- *Navigating Breast Cancer: A Guide for the Newly Diagnosed*

- *100 Questions & Answers About Advanced and Metastatic Breast Cancer*

- *Johns Hopkins Patients' Guide to Breast Cancer*

- *Kids Speak Out About Breast Cancer*

FOR YOU AS A PROFESSIONAL

- *The Johns Hopkins Breast Cancer Handbook for Health Care Professionals*

ORGANIZATIONS OF BENEFIT TO YOU AND YOUR PATIENTS

American Cancer Society (ACS)

800-227-2345, www.cancer.org

The ACS offers financial guidance to patients and their families. Type *financial and legal matters* into the search box to find brochures such as "How to Find a Financial Professional Sensitive to Cancer Issues" and "Coping Financially with the Loss of a Loved One." The ACS also offers programs such as Look Good, Feel Better, which provides guidance in how to wear scarves, hats, and turbans as well as makeup tips that can help patients who are undergoing chemotherapy and experiencing hair loss and skin changes. The ACS can also provide free transportation for cancer treatments through their Road to Recovery program. They also have a program called Reach to Recovery that offers the opportunity for a newly diagnosed breast cancer patient to speak with a breast cancer survivor. Also read online about the funding they have provided for patient navigation programs with a special focus on laypersons serving in a navigation role.

breastcancer.org

breastcancer.org is a nonprofit organization dedicated to providing the most reliable, complete, and up-to-date information about breast cancer. Their mission is to help women and their loved ones make sense of the complex medical and personal information about breast cancer so they can make the best decisions for their lives. Their Web site contains excellent, easy-to-understand educational information about breast health and breast cancer for patients and families. They also have online seminars and phone conferences to bring breast cancer patients and survivors together on topics of interest such as sexual dysfunction caused by hormonal therapy, fertility issues, managing side effects of chemotherapy, lymphedema, and information about new data from clinical trials results.

Cancer Information Service of the National Cancer Institute

800-4-CANCER, www.cancer.gov

This organization provides information about all types of cancer including excellent information about breast cancer, what it is, how it is treated, and where various treatment options are provided. You can request free information by calling the toll-free number. Visit their Web site for information about patient navigation. They are a major grant resource for navigation programs.

Komen for the Cure

National help line 800-IM-AWARE
www.breastcancerinfo.com, www.komen.org

This is a national volunteer organization seeking to eradicate breast cancer as a life-threatening disease, by working through local chapters and the Race for the Cure, events held in more than 110 cities. The foundation is the largest private funder of breast cancer research in the United States. The Komen Alliance is a comprehensive program for the research, education, diagnosis, and treatment of breast disease. You and your patients will find educational information on their Web site. It also provides funding to some breast centers in support of navigation and addressing the needs of the underserved.

Mothers Supporting Daughters with Breast Cancer (MSDBC)

410-778-1982,

msdbc@verizon.net, www.mothersdaughters.org

This is a national nonprofit organization dedicated to providing support to mothers who have daughters diagnosed with breast cancer. This organization offers a free "mother's handbook" and "daughter's companion booklet" that provides basic information about breast cancer and its treatment as well as some recommended constructive ways for mothers to provide support physically, emotionally, financially, and spiritually. The organization also "matches" mothers as mother volunteers across the country based on the daughter's (patient's) clinical picture, age at time of diagnosis, and anticipated treatment plan.

Network of Strength

800-221-2141 (24-hour national hotline),

800-986-9505 (24-hour hotline in Spanish)

info@y-me.org, www.y-me.org

Network of Strength (previously known as Y-Me) is committed to providing information and support to anyone who has been touched by breast cancer. The services listed on their Web site include a national hotline for women needing emotional support; kid's corner; referral information for approved mammography facilities near you;

public education workshops where you will find a listing of upcoming events; teen programs where you can order a video specifically for teenage girls to learn about breast cancer awareness; and a resource library that provides information about treatment modalities. Your patients will also find a special interactive feature on the Web site called "Breast Cancer Coach." This is a teaching tool to educate patients about breast cancer and how to translate information contained within their pathology report. (I serve as the breast cancer coach.)

Young Survival Coalition

155 6th Avenue, 10th Floor, New York, NY 10013
212-206-6610, info@youngsurvival.org,
www.youngsurvival.org

The Young Survival Coalition (YSC) is the only international, nonprofit network of breast cancer survivors and supporters dedicated to the concerns and issues that are unique to young women and breast cancer. Through action, advocacy, and awareness, the YSC seeks to educate the medical, research, breast cancer, and legislative communities and to persuade them to address breast cancer in women 40 and under. The YSC also serves as a point of contact for young women living with breast cancer. They offer quarterly conferences to educate young women about issues that are specific to their needs, such as fertility preservation, long-term bone health, genetics counseling and testing, cognitive functioning as a side effect of chemotherapy, reconstruction options, and other topics of particular interest to a young woman dealing with breast cancer or having survived breast cancer. The YCS oftentimes hold their conferences in collaboration with Living Beyond Breast Cancer, another nonprofit organization dedicated to educating and supporting breast cancer survivors.

ADDITIONAL FINANCIAL AND LEGAL RESOURCES

Accompanying any serious illness are questions and concerns related to expenses incurred as a result of treatment, health insurance questions that can be overwhelming for patients to try to understand or resolve alone, and sometimes even legal questions related to employment or financial matters. Below is a list of national resources to aid you in addressing these types of concerns for your patients:

Cancer Care, Inc.
212-302-2400, 800-813-HOPE
info@cancercare.org, www.cancercare.org

Cancer Care is a national nonprofit organization that provides free, professional assistance to people with any type of cancer and to their families. This organization offers education, one-on-one counseling, financial assistance for nonmedical expenses and referrals to community services.

National Coalition for Cancer Survivorship (NCCS)
301-650-8868, 877-NCSS-YES
info@ccansearch.org, www.cansearch.org

This network of independent groups and individuals provide information and resources about cancer support, advocacy, and quality-of-life issues as well as helps cancer patients deal with insurance or job discrimination and other related legal matters.

Patient Advocate Foundation

800-532-5274, www.patientadvocate.org/report.php

866-512-3861, www.copays.org

The National Financial Resources Guidebook for Patients is a state-by-state directory of programs and services that assists patients with housing, utilities, food, and transportation to medical treatment. In addition, PAF helps insured patients who qualify to access copay assistance from pharmaceutical companies through its Co-Pay Relief Program.

PHARMACEUTICAL ASSISTANCE PROGRAMS

For a list of drug and patient assistance programs go to www.curetoday.com/assistance_programs.

ADDITIONAL RESOURCES AND PROFESSIONAL ORGANIZATIONS OF SPECIFIC BENEFIT TO BREAST CENTER PATIENT NAVIGATORS

Having the opportunity to network with others and learn from their experiences as well as exchange information and ideas can truly be beneficial to you and your future patients. There is no glory in reinventing the wheel. Though each breast center is unique, there are some similarities within their organizational structures as well as probably the overall missions and purposes. Take advantage of meeting other navigators at national conferences, regional meetings, and online. Below are some specific resources for you that are worthy of your time and participation.

PROFESSIONAL ORGANIZATIONS OF BENEFIT
TO NURSE NAVIGATORS

You will benefit from networking with others who are performing similar roles and functions like yourself. There are several organizations worthy of your time and membership participation. They are listed for you below and provide a wealth of opportunities for networking, exchange of ideas that have worked elsewhere (to prevent you from having to reinvent the wheel), and even opportunities for you to become certified as a nurse navigator in a breast center. Adding such credentials to your name can benefit you when seeking a promotion, increase in salary, or simply because you want to demonstrate to your patients that you are very knowledgeable about the field of breast cancer.

National Consortium of Breast Centers Certification Program for Navigators
 www.breastcare.org
 www.bpnc.org/index.cfm

The consortium, which consists of more than 900 breast centers nationally (and internationally) offers membership opportunities for breast center navigators as well as an opportunity to become certified as a navigator. In an effort to minimize variances in a breast patient's continuum of care and the definition and function of a breast patient navigator providing care within that continuum,

NCBC developed a breast care continuum matrix. The Breast Patient Navigation Matrix offers a model for continuity in a breast patient's care, which can be adopted and modified by facilities providing breast care and cancer services.

The matrix identifies the navigation stages within the breast patient's continuum of care. Each navigation stage begins and ends with the patient as the focus. It further identifies the integrated navigation team member(s) who may be called upon for assistance in each navigation stage. Integrated team members include medically credentialed professionals, nonmedically credentialed professionals, consultants, and volunteers. The navigation stages are separated into two sets: breast imaging stages and breast cancer diagnosis and treatment stages.

Based upon the navigation stages in the matrix, the breast patient navigator's role and function is defined. The breast patient navigator's expected performance and knowledge is identified for each navigation stage. Thus a set of activities and associated knowledge are linked with each navigation stage.

This model allows the breast patient navigator to assist patients with (1) understanding the continuum of their care, (2) knowing who and how to contact the appropriate individual on staff for various services and support throughout their stages of care, (3) identifying resources available to them at various times as needed, and (4) empowering them to become informed participants in their breast health or cancer care program.

To set standards of achievement based upon the professional's role; enhance patient safety, quality of care, and delivery of services; and recognize professionals who advance beyond basic knowledge in a field of specialty, the National Consortium of Breast Centers developed a Breast Patient Navigation Certification.

Certification is offered annually at their national conference in March each year as well as regionally during other times of the year. For more information, visit their Web site at www.breastcare.org. I serve on the task force that developed their certification program and am a speaker at the national meeting and at some of the regional certification program conferences.

The Breast Patient Navigation Certification examination is based upon the role of a breast patient navigator and the Breast Patient Navigation Matrix. A peer review team of breast patient navigators, selected by discipline, facility and program type, and geographical area participated in the role and matrix demarcation. The Breast Patient Navigation Certification examination reflects the knowledge and skills a breast patient navigator should understand in order to successfully navigate a breast patient through the breast health/cancer continuum of care. Due to advancements in care processes, treatments, and technology, the examination is continually reviewed to reflect these advancements.

You need to have some navigation experience under your belt before considering taking the certification exam.

Certification continuation must be demonstrated annually through professional education and documented performance.

The Academy of Oncology Nurse Navigators (AONN)

www.aonnonline.org

This is a national specialty organization dedicated to improving patient care and quality of life by defining, enhancing, and promoting the role of oncology nurse navigators for patients and their families, as well as cancer centers, hospitals, and community practices.

The mission of AONN is to provide a network for oncology nurses, nurse navigators, practice managers, patient care coordinators, and nursing administrators to better manage the complexities of the cancer care continuum focused on improving the treatment and quality of life of patients. The vision of AONN is to increase the role of and access to oncology nurse navigators, so that all cancer patients may benefit from their guidance, insight, and personal advocacy.

This organization, which consists of more than 1500 members (as of November 2009), was founded in May 2009. Through the information provided by this academy, oncology nurse navigators have access to vast resources on patient care, continuing education, and dialogues with their peers. The AONN Web site provides educational information including articles authored by oncology nurse navigators that provide examples of how to approach a particular navigation issue as well as ongoing education related to cancer diagnosis, treatment, survivorship, navigation, and other topics applicable for an oncology nurse navigator audience. You will find articles written by me monthly. The AONN also holds annual conferences for oncology nurse navigators, which a great opportunity for professionals like yourself to come together, learn, and network with one another.

SOFTWARE DESIGNED TO HELP TRACK PATIENTS AND PRODUCE REPORTS ON NAVIGATION PERFORMANCE

Priority Consult Breast Care

www.priorityconsult.com

Priority Consult Breast Care is a customizable and comprehensive breast patient navigation and clinical tracking computer program. Supporting both nurse and nonnurse patient navigators, the program assists breast center staff in directing and following a patient from initial screening or diagnostic imaging, to biopsy and pathology, through treatment and follow-up. Navigators responsible for patients at a particular stage in care benefit from a notification of a patient's status as well as a prompt when an action is scheduled to occur. This is done through the use of a sophisticated queuing and alert system that mirrors the breast care continuum. The queuing system enables breast center staff to view the status and next step of every active patient within the program. Information regarding a patient at a particular stage is gathered and stored within the Priority Consult Breast Care system. The information is used to create treatment summaries for members of the tumor board. Once a patient has been presented before the tumor board, a navigator can enter into the system the recommended treatment plan and use the information to help forecast, in an easy-to-understand visual form, what the patient can expect during the course of her treatment.

After a patient has been tracked through her treatment phase of care, a navigator can once again use the program to forecast a patient's next step—her survivorship plan. Custom survivorship planning documents are built into the software program and when generated, take into account the treatment a patient has received. Ongoing follow-up is managed through a queuing system that alerts breast center staff when it is time to complete scheduled follow-up. The software is also designed to report breast center clinical quality and operational efficiency indicators as laid out by such organizations as the National Quality Measures for Breast Centers. For more information regarding Priority Consult Breast Care visit www.priorityconsult.com.

CREATING YOUR OWN INTERNAL AND EXTERNAL RESOURCE LIST

Resources

Name	:	*Mary Smith*
Title	:	*Social Worker*
Phone	:	*5-8989*
Fax	:	*5-8988*

1. *Apply for medical assistance*
2. *Pharmacy discount*
3. *Taxi voucher for transportation*

Name	:	_____
Title	:	_____
Phone	:	_____
Fax	:	_____

1. _____
2. _____
3. _____

Name	:	_____
Title	:	_____
Phone	:	_____
Fax	:	_____

1. _____
2. _____
3. _____

Name	:	_____
Title	:	_____
Phone	:	_____
Fax	:	_____

1. _____
2. _____
3. _____

External Contact List

Resources

Name : *John Jones*

Address : *ACS Office*

1. *Road to Recovery*
2. *Free Wigs*
3. *Look Good Feel Great*

Phone : *555-5555*

Fax : *555-5555*

Name : _____

Address : _____

_____

1. _____
2. _____
3. _____

Phone : _____

Fax : _____

Name : _____

Address : _____

_____

1. _____
2. _____
3. _____

Phone : _____

Fax : _____

Name : _____

Address : _____

_____

1. _____
2. _____
3. _____

Phone : _____

Fax : _____

PATIENT NAVIGATOR OUTREACH AND CHRONIC DISEASE PREVENTION ACT OF 2005

PUBLIC LAW 109–18
109TH CONGRESS

An Act

To amend the Public Health Service Act to authorize a demonstration grant program to provide patient navigator services to reduce barriers and improve health care outcomes, and for other purposes.

Be it enacted by the Senate and House of Representatives of the United States of America in Congress assembled,

SECTION 1. SHORT TITLE

This Act may be cited as the "Patient Navigator Outreach and Chronic Disease Prevention Act of 2005".

SEC. 2. PATIENT NAVIGATOR GRANTS

Subpart V of part D of title III of the Public Health Service Act (42 U.S.C. 256) is amended by adding at the end the following:

"SEC. 340A. PATIENT NAVIGATOR GRANTS

"(a) GRANTS.—The Secretary, acting through the Administrator of the Health Resources and Services Administration, may make grants to eligible entities for the development and operation of demonstration programs to provide patient navigator services to improve health care outcomes. The Secretary shall coordinate with, and ensure the participation of, the Indian Health Service, the National Cancer Institute, the Office of Rural Health Policy, and such other offices and agencies as deemed appropriate by the Secretary, regarding the design and evaluation of the demonstration programs.

"(b) USE OF FUNDS.—The Secretary shall require each recipient of a grant under this section to use the grant to recruit, assign, train, and employ patient navigators who have direct knowledge of the communities they serve to facilitate the care of individuals, including by performing each of the following duties:

"(1) Acting as contacts, including by assisting in the coordination of health care services and provider referrals, for individuals who are seeking prevention or early detection services for, or who following a screening or early detection service are found to have a symptom, abnormal finding, or diagnosis of, cancer or other chronic disease.

"(2) Facilitating the involvement of community organizations in assisting individuals who are at risk for or who have cancer or other chronic diseases to receive better access to high-quality health care services (such as by creating partnerships with patient advocacy groups, charities, health care centers, community hospice centers, other health care providers, or other organizations in the targeted community).

"(3) Notifying individuals of clinical trials and, on request, facilitating enrollment of eligible individuals in these trials.

"(4) Anticipating, identifying, and helping patients to overcome barriers within the health care system to ensure prompt diagnostic and treatment resolution of an abnormal finding of cancer or other chronic disease.

"(5) Coordinating with the relevant health insurance ombudsman programs to provide information to individuals who are at risk for or who have cancer or other chronic diseases about health coverage, including private insurance, health care savings accounts, and other publicly funded programs (such as Medicare, Medicaid, health programs operated by the Department of Veterans Affairs or the Department of Defense, the State children's health insurance program, and any private or governmental prescription assistance programs).

"(6) Conducting ongoing outreach to health disparity populations, including the uninsured, rural populations, and other medically under-served populations, in addition to assisting other individuals who are at risk for or who have cancer or other chronic diseases to seek preventative care.

"(c) PROHIBITIONS.—

"(1) REFERRAL FEES.—The Secretary shall require each recipient of a grant under this section to prohibit any patient navigator providing ser-vices under the grant from accepting any referral fee, kickback, or other thing of value in return for referring an individual to a particular health care provider.

"(2) LEGAL FEES AND COSTS.—The Sec-retary shall prohibit the use of any grant funds received under this section to pay any fees or costs resulting from any litigation, arbitration, media-tion, or other proceeding to resolve a legal dispute.

"(d) GRANT PERIOD.—

"(1) IN GENERAL.—Subject to paragraphs (2) and (3), the Secretary may award grants under this section for periods of not more than 3 years.

"(2) EXTENSIONS.—Subject to paragraph (3), the Secretary may extend the period of a grant under this section. Each such extension shall be for a period of not more than 1 year.

"(3) LIMITATIONS ON GRANT PERIOD.—In carrying out this section, the Secretary—

"(A) shall ensure that the total period of a grant does not exceed 4 years; and

"(B) may not authorize any grant period ending after September 30, 2010.

"(e) APPLICATION.—

"(1) IN GENERAL.—To seek a grant under this section, an eligible entity shall submit an application to the Secretary in such form, in such manner, and containing such information as the Secretary may require.

"(2) CONTENTS.—At a minimum, the Secretary shall require each such application to outline how the eligible entity will establish baseline measures and benchmarks that meet the Secretary's requirements to evaluate program outcomes.

"(f) UNIFORM BASELINE MEASURES.—The Secretary shall establish uniform baseline measures in order to properly evaluate the impact of the demonstration projects under this section.

"(g) PREFERENCE.—In making grants under this section, the Secretary shall give preference to eligible entities that demonstrate in their applications plans to utilize patient navigator services to overcome significant barriers in order to improve health care outcomes in their respective communities.

"(h) DUPLICATION OF SERVICES.—An eligible entity that is receiving Federal funds for activities described in subsection (b) on the date on which the entity submits an application under subsection (e) may not receive a grant under this section unless the entity can demonstrate that amounts received under the grant will be utilized to expand services or provide new services to individuals who would not otherwise be served.

"(i) COORDINATION WITH OTHER PROGRAMS.—The Secretary shall ensure coordination of the demonstration grant program under this section with existing authorized programs in order to facilitate access to high-quality health care services.

"(j) STUDY; REPORTS.—

"(1) FINAL REPORT BY SECRETARY.—Not later than 6 months after the completion of the demonstration grant program under this section, the Secretary shall conduct a study of the results of the program and submit to the Congress a report on such results that includes the following:

"(A) An evaluation of the program outcomes, including—

"(i) quantitative analysis of baseline and benchmark measures; and

"(ii) aggregate information about the patients served and program activities.

"(B) Recommendations on whether patient navigator programs could be used to improve patient outcomes in other public health areas.

"(2) INTERIM REPORTS BY SECRETARY.—
The Secretary may provide interim reports to
the Congress on the demonstration grant program under this section at such intervals as the
Secretary determines to be appropriate.

"(3) REPORTS BY GRANTEES.—The Secretary may require grant recipients under this
section to submit interim and final reports on
grant program outcomes.

"(k) RULE OF CONSTRUCTION.—This section
shall not be construed to authorize funding for the
delivery of health care services (other than the patient
navigator duties listed in subsection (b)).

"(l) DEFINITIONS.—In this section:

"(1) The term 'eligible entity' means a public
or nonprofit private health center (including a
Federally qualified health center (as that term
is defined in section 1861(aa)(4) of the Social
Security Act)), a health facility operated by or pursuant to a contract with the Indian Health Service,
a hospital, a cancer center, a rural health clinic, an
academic health center, or a nonprofit entity that
enters into a partnership or coordinates referrals
with such a center, clinic, facility, or hospital to
provide patient navigator services.

"(2) The term 'health disparity population'
means a population that, as determined by
the Secretary, has a significant disparity in the
overall rate of disease incidence, prevalence,
morbidity, mortality, or survival rates as

compared to the health status of the general population.

"(3) The term 'patient navigator' means an individual who has completed a training program approved by the Secretary to perform the duties listed in subsection (b).

"(m) AUTHORIZATION OF APPROPRIATIONS.—

"(1) IN GENERAL.—To carry out this section, there are authorized to be appropriated $2,000,000 for fiscal year 2006, $5,000,000 for fiscal year 2007, $8,000,000 for fiscal year 2008, $6,500,000 for fiscal year 2009, and $3,500,000 for fiscal year 2010.

"(2) AVAILABILITY.—The amounts appropriated pursuant to paragraph (1) shall remain available for obligation through the end of fiscal year 2010.".

Approved June 29, 2005.

INDEX

sharing of resources, 80
social worker, 59, 60, 70, 71,
  75–76
software for patient navigation,
  35–36, 122–23
stages of disease
  at diagnosis, 80, 82,
    87, 92
  navigator's knowledge
    of treatment
    considerations, 22
success of program.
    See performance
    measurement
support groups, 27
support services, use of, 79.
    See also Red Devils
    patient services
surgical consultation, 41, 42,
  60–61
surgical treatment
  myths about, 90, 93
  navigator's knowledge, 21
  patient compliance, 101
  preoperative tests and
    appointment, 44–45
  reviewing with patient, 42
surveying consumers, 90
survival rates, 80
survivor volunteers
  Johns Hopkins program, 96,
    97, 98, 100
  as mentors, 3
  as navigators, 70
survivorship plan, 22, 36, 56–58,
  122–23
system barriers, 16, 23, 79

time allocation, 82
time delays (lags)
  performance measurement,
    80, 105*t*
  reducing, 26, 27, 32–35,
    95–96, 98

tracking the patient
  developing and implementing
    system, 77
  post-surgical treatment and
    survivorship plan, 52, 53,
    55, 57–58
  screening through surgical
    postop appointment,
    38–39, 41, 47, 49
  software, 35–36, 122–23
transportation
  Johns Hopkins and, 96, 99
  lack of, as barrier to care, 3, 13,
    16, 23
  performance measurement
    and, 79, 81
  providing access to, 52, 78
treatment plan
  burden on patients, 14–15
  guiding patient through, 2, 4
  navigation software and, 36,
    122–23
  patient compliance, 101
  patient confusion, 89, 92
  patient education about, 92, 99
  reviewing options with
    patient, 42, 43
  time delays, 26, 27, 32–35
    See also adherence to
    treatment plan
tumor-site models for patient
    navigation (traditional),
    61–62, 63*t*, 65–66

UM (utilization management),
    8–9, 11*t*, 12
underserved populations, 13
  barriers to cancer screening
    and care, 13, 15–16
  community outreach, 62, 75.
    See also community
    outreach
  screening mammograms, 62,
    75, 79, 96